Enzyme Therapy Basics

Powerful Remedies for Women

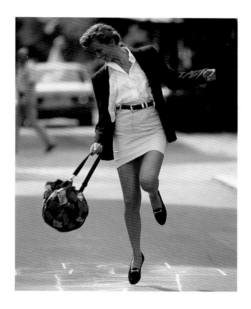

Friedrich W. Dittmar, M.D.
&
Jutta Wellmann

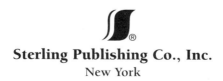

Sterling Publishing Co., Inc.
New York

This book is by no means intended as a self-help guide. Female disorders, in particular, always require a physician to establish their cause and to help in deciding on the right treatment.

Library of Congress Cataloging-in-Publication Data

Dittmar, Friedrich-W.
   [Enzyme Aktivstoffe für Frauen. English]
   Enzyme therapy basics : powerful remedies for women / Friedrich-W. Dittmar & Jutta Wellmann.
      p.   cm.
   ISBN 0-8069-2031-9
   1. Women—Diseases—Nutritional aspects. 2.Enzymes—Therapeutic use. 3. Dietary
supplements. I. Wellmann, Jutta. II. Title.
   RA778.D5813 1999
   615'.35'082—dc21   99-37531
                                                                                                                            CIP

Translation edited by Laurel Ornitz
Photos and Illustrations: APE: p. 17, 21, 43, 77; AKG: p. 97 (Lessing); All over: p. 45 (Kröner); Bavaria: front cover (Stock image), p. 32 (The Telegraph), p. 81 (Seward), p. 108 (TCL), p. 144 (Lorentis); Gerlind Bruhn: p. 126; Franz Faltermaier: p. 146; G+J, Bokelberg: back cover, p. 9; GMF, Bonn: p. 8; Stefan Gustavus: p. 115; Fotodesign Hesselmann: p. 54; hohes C, Food Professionals: p. 106; IDM, Bonn: p. 29; Image Bank: front flap (top and middle), p. 2 (top), p. 3 (left), p. 11 (Wolf), p. 19, p. 25 (de Lossy), p. 35 (Wolf), p. 40 (Redfearn), p. 67 (Bistram), p. 72 (Regine M.); Info Banane, Ketchum PR: p. 150; Ulla Kimmig: p. 111; Klafs Saunabau: p. 129; Susanne Kracke: p. 133; Köllnflockenwerke: pp. 14-15; Mauritius: p. 2 (bottom), p. 13, p. 39 (Hubatka), p. 65, p. 104; Pictor: p. 113; Thomas v. Salomon: pp. 91, 92, 112; Reiner Schmitz: back flap (top), p. 3 (left), pp. 7, 26, 31, 37, 47, 99, 121, 124, 141 (styling: Jeanette Heerwagen); Christophe Schneider: pp. 62, 101, 114, 135; Teubner: p. 142; Tony Stone: front flap (bottom), back inside flap, p. 4, p. 59 (Correz), p. 61 (Ayres), p. 75 (Madison), p. 85 (Coates), p. 89 (Herholdt), p. 103 (Bisell), p. 118 (Madison), p. 137 (Harvey), p. 147 (Shonnard), p. 149 (Correz); Transglobe: back flap (middle), p. 49, p. 71; Wunsch: front inside flap; ZEFA: p. 116 (Barton).
Our thanks to: Mr. Wolfgang Glaser, for his expert advice;

10 9 8 7 6 5 4 3 2 1

Published by Sterling Publishing Company, Inc.
387 Park Avenue South, New York, N.Y. 10016
First published in Germany under the title *Enzyme: Aktivstoffe
für Frauen* and © 1996 by Gräfe und Unser Verlag GmbH, Munich
Translation © 2000 by Sterling Publishing Company, Inc.
Distributed in Canada by Sterling Publishing
C/o Canadian Manda Group, One Atlantic Avenue, Suite 105
Toronto, Ontario, Canada M6K 3E7
Distributed in Great Britain and Europe by Cassell PLC
Wellington House, 125 Strand, London WC2R 0BB, England
Distributed in Australia by Capricorn Link (Australia) Pty Ltd.
P.O. Box 6651, Baulkham Hills, Business Centre, NSW 2153, Australia

Printed in China
All rights reserved

Sterling ISBN 0-8069-2031-9

The Mind-Body Problem
  Rebecca Newberger Goldstein

new/ 36 arguments for the
        existence of God - a work
           of fiction

The Hidden Brain: How Our
minds elect Presidents Control
markets, wage Wars & Save our
lives   by Shankar Vedantam

Barney Frank: The Story of America's
  Only Left-Handed, Gay, Jewish
  Congressman
          by Stewart E. Weisberg

Day Out of Days - Sam Shepherd 25⁰⁰
   Collection of Stories

(D.H. Lawrence —) Concerning E.H. Forrester
(melville)   by Frank Kermode

          /over

<u>Children Who Changed the World</u> by ~~Leonard S. Marcus~~

→ <u>Marching for Freedom: Walk Together, Children, and Don't you Grow Weary.</u> by Elizabeth Partridge — Winter + Spring of 1965 the March on Montgomery that Crystallized Congressional Support for Voters' rights legislation.

Her prev. books for young adults (10 + up) — biographies: Woodie Guthrie, John Lennon + Dorothea Lange

<u>One Crazy Summer</u> by Rita Williams garcia
(ages 9-12)

Contents

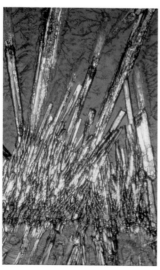

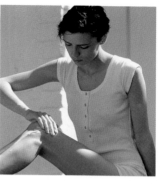

Contents

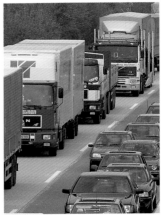

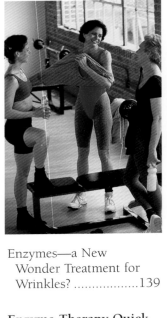

Preface

Over the last few years, there has been a growing interest in enzymes as effective remedies, especially for women. The tiny enzyme molecules have numerous, surprising effects. They accelerate the healing process following many forms of gynecological treatment and thus prevent complications and later aftereffects. But this isn't all. They are now used in the treatment of breast diseases, lymphatic edema, vein complaints, and many other disorders. Particularly where female ailments are concerned, there is hardly one that would not benefit from the use of enzyme treatment. Enzymes are now also making a name for themselves in aftercare following surgery and in childbirth, and they even help in the treatment of minor injuries, blocked sinuses, and stiff muscles.

- Enzyme therapies are reported to be amazingly successful. You too can make good use of the healing powers of enzymes. In this guide, we show you how you can strengthen your own enzyme system effectively with specific preparations as well as through your diet and by means of sufficient exercise.
- It is our view that enzymes are today's gentle route to better health, without the fear of side effects, for you and your family.

Most disorders, but particularly those that affect women, will benefit from enzyme treatment. And we are not making an empty promise when we say that enzymes will also improve your fitness and do wonders for your looks. More and more cosmetic products contain enzymes and their helpers, coenzymes. New scientific research shows again and again how important these biological substances are for an attractive appearance. When your body is armed with enzymes, you are less susceptible to stress, suffer less harm from the growing number of toxins in the environment, and are protected from premature aging of the skin—as well as from more serious problems such as heart attacks and cancer.

Friedrich W. Dittmar, M.D., is the head of the gynecological clinic at the district hospital in Starnberg, Germany. **Jutta Wellmann** is a medical journalist.

Enzymes—the Spark of Life

You can't see them, but enzymes are everywhere. Each and every cell in our bodies produces them, and they are contained in a great variety of food. All of these tiny enzyme molecules know exactly where they are supposed to go to work. They are the sparks without which the engine of life will not start.

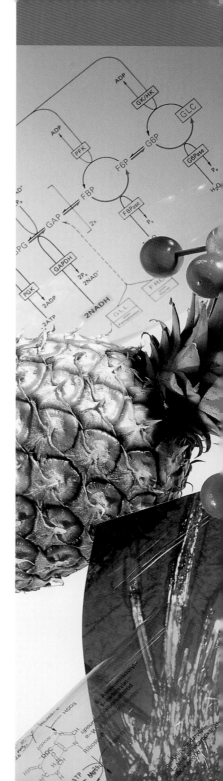

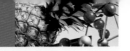

The Source of Vitality

Have you ever sat at the breakfast table and thought about enzymes? Probably not. But enzymes are everywhere. Without them, the dough for bread would not rise. We wouldn't be able to digest a single bite of food or absorb any of the nutrients in our food if enzymes weren't there to help.

Enzymes in Everyday Life

The enzymes in bread, rolls, and other baked goods make sure that the dough rises and a nice crust develops, and that the finished product looks appetizing and has the same great taste every day. Food chemists call these enzymes amylase, protease, lipoxygenase, and phospholipase.

The dairy industry has come to depend on enzymes too. Cheese production, in particular, uses a protein-splitting enzyme called rennin, which is found in the stomachs of calves. The taste and the quality of cheese depend mainly

Did you know that you encounter enzymes wherever you go at the market? Meat, cheese, fruit juices, alcohol—they all contain enzymes! Without them, nothing much would happen in food production.

It takes a multitude of tiny enzymes to turn water, flour, and yeast into delicious bread.

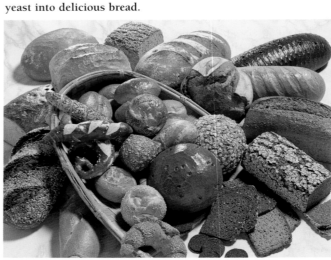

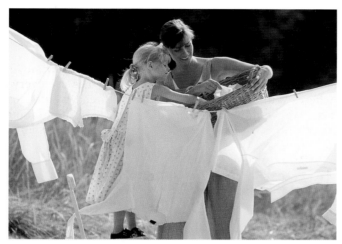

Only if you wash your laundry at low temperatures can enzymes help to remove protein and grease stains.

Tip
When you buy laundry detergents, make sure that they contain enzymes. These detergents will help you to save money by cleaning effectively even at lower temperatures, and they are also kinder to the environment.

on which combination of enzymes took part at a particular time during the ripening process.

There are no longer enough enzymes available from animal sources to supply cheese production worldwide. However, natural enzymes can now be synthesized in laboratories with the help of microorganisms.

Enzymes also play an important role in fermentation. Without them, the fermentation of fruit juices would take much longer. They are also responsible for making many foods the way we expect them to be. Without these little biological helpers, red wine wouldn't be red, meat wouldn't be tender, and desserts wouldn't be sweet.

Powerful Whitening Agents

Some people have only become aware of enzymes since they were added to laundry detergents, with the promise of leaving our clothes the cleanest we have ever seen them. The enzymes at work in these biological detergents are called protease. They destroy the proteins that are the main component of stains by literally consuming them. But they also fight other substances that they encounter in

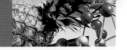

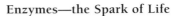

the washing machine. Greasy stains, for example, are dissolved even at low temperatures.

Enzymes for laundry detergents, just like those found in food, are manufactured in laboratories using biotechnical processes. Unlike phosphates and other solvents, they are a hundred percent biodegradable and therefore go a long way toward protecting the environment.

How Enzymes Were Discovered

Enzymes were discovered more or less by accident. The French chemist and bacteriologist Louis Pasteur (1822 to 1895) was conducting ongoing research into what substances play a role in fermentation and putrefaction. One day he was approached by a student of his with a private concern: His father was a vintner and had run into trouble with his harvest that summer. For some strange reason, the juice from the grapes had turned into an undrinkable, murky liquid instead of wine. Pasteur was eager to help the family and agreed to look into the cause of the disaster.

At the time, yeast was the fermenting agent for wine. Fermentation was triggered, it was assumed, by a biological substance that was consequently called "ferment." Pasteur examined both the unsuccessful and a successful product of fermentation under the microscope and in both cases discovered live cell cultures. He then rushed to tell his colleagues in the scientific community his astounding discoveries: the existence of a second ferment and the fact that both ferments were linked to living cells (in the case of wine, these are yeast cells).

Today, a distinction between ferment and enzymes is no longer made, as both terms stand for the same thing—namely, the protein molecules necessary to start numerous reactions in nature and in the human body.

A Dispute among Scientists

Pasteur's colleagues, however, did not believe that the ferment always depended on live cells. For instance, other biochemists found ferment in grain where it splits up starch without the existence of live cells. The dispute raged on for years, with the scientists eventually settling on a compromise: The substances coupled with live cells would continue to be called "ferment," whereas the substances that were independent of live cells would thereafter be called "enzymes."

10

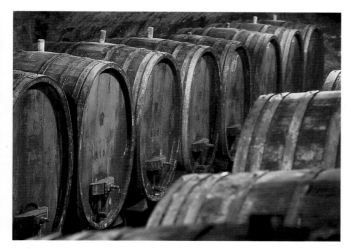

Although wine has been produced for thousands of years, the role of enzymes in the fermentation process was discovered only about a hundred years ago.

At the beginning of enzyme research, there was a long-lasting dispute among scientists regarding the fermentation of wine.

Decades later, in 1897, an unknown chemist from Munich by the name of Eduard Buchner discovered—again by accident—that alcoholic fermentation does in fact work with enzymes alone and without live yeast cells. For this insight, he was later awarded the Nobel prize. It had finally been established that enzymes and ferment were exactly the same—for once, the great Pasteur had been mistaken.

Enzymes at the Beginning of All Life

The development of human life, or any life at all for that matter, would have been impossible without enzymes. They are essential ingredients for all plant, animal, and human life. Scientists today know that up to 40,000 enzymes are involved in all biological processes on earth, and 4,000 of them have been researched in some detail. Without these tiny protein molecules, life would not be possible. In the body, enzymes turn food into energy and enable cells to breathe and divide. They allow the body to utilize substances essential to life, such as oxygen, protein, fat, and

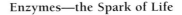

carbohydrates. Other enzymes make sure that our bodies excrete those waste products and toxins found in food that they are unable to use. Thousands of different types of enzyme are at work in the human body all the time.

Working Where They Are Needed—and Fast

From a biochemical point of view, enzymes are catalysts, which means that even small amounts of enzymes will accelerate chemical reactions. Consequently, they are found in the body wherever fast action is necessary—for example, in supplying the body with oxygen. Enzymes ensure that the iron in the red blood cells quickly binds the oxygen we breathe in from the air. Without these enzymes, we would suffocate. The red blood cells then transport the oxygen from the lungs to the various organs, where other enzymes help to make the oxygen accessible as quickly as possible. Enzymes therefore prevent a large-scale dying of cells and consequently illness.

They Are So Tiny . . .

Enzymes are so small that they can't be detected with a normal microscope. Scientists have still not quite grasped their structure. These microscopic substances form long and complex chains of proteins (amino acid chains), the function of which is not yet fully known, because it is only a short section of the chain that performs the necessary work. Enzymes are composed of proteins that the body produces itself. The vast majority of enzymes needed in the body are produced in the body's cells.

The approximately 50,000 genes of a cell dictate the structure of the enzyme. The actual component of the cell where the enzymes are produced is the ribosome. Once an enzyme has been assembled from various protein particles, it is sent through a kind of quality control to ensure that only fully functioning enzymes are dispatched to work.

. . . and Yet So Powerful

Each type of enzyme is assigned a specific task. Enzymes can be divided roughly into two groups. The first group acts

Native Americans already knew how to use the healing power of enzymes. A chief by the name of Rolling Thunder is reported to have treated his warriors' wounds by applying raw meat. The enzymes in the meat accelerated the healing process.

inside a cell to ensure that it receives all it needs to live. Numerous safeguards prevent faulty enzymes from delivering wrong or harmful substances to a cell. The gateway to the cell is well guarded and difficult to find. It is located in the outer layer of the cell, the membrane, and has only a few openings. Each opening has a guard checking carefully whether or not the delivered nutrients comply with the quality standards of the cell. The second group of enzymes

Enzymes (here, seen under an electronic microscope) are among the busiest molecules in the body. A single enzyme can spring into action up to 36 million times a minute.

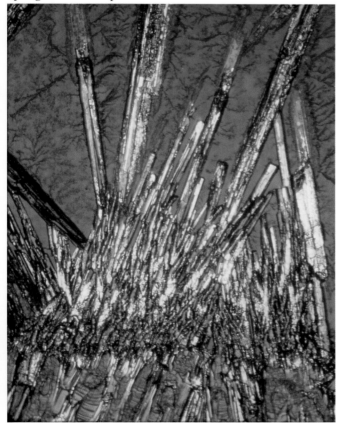

Practically all processes in the body are powered by enzymes—from breathing and digestion to the formation of muscles and the production of hormones.

acts outside the cell and is responsible for splitting up food and transporting the usable parts to the cells. Other enzymes in this group, as mentioned earlier, are responsible for the oxygen supply to the body.

Enzymes in the Mouth, the Stomach, and the Digestive Tract

A cell doesn't have much use for a piece of bread, even if it is chewed well. It is far too big to be absorbed by a tiny cell. Food therefore has to be split into the individual nutrients of which it consists. This is done by enzymes. There are special digestive enzymes called amylase, which are contained in the saliva, where they start their digestive work. Saliva also contains other useful enzymes that destroy harmful substances found in food, such as bacteria. The amylase get straight to work in the mouth, separating sugar and starch molecules from the food. The chewed food then continues to the stomach, where it is attacked by gastric acid.

The aggressive nature of the gastric acid destroys the last remaining harmful substances in the food (bacteria and viruses). But it also destroys the amylase, whose digestive work thus comes to an abrupt stop. Gastric acid eradicates all protein molecules, including enzymes, with the exception of one: pepsin, which resists the acid. The amylase split up carbohydrates, whereas pepsin splits up proteins. Depending on whether or not we have eaten food that is easily digested, it takes up to 12 hours for gastric acid and pepsin to complete their digestive work.

Tip
Always chew your food slowly and thoroughly, because this allows the enzymes in the mouth to do optimal work. Have you ever noticed how bread, when you chew it for a long time, develops a sweet flavor? This is a sure sign that the enzymes in your saliva are doing their job.

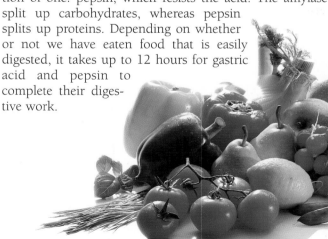

From Menu to Molecule

Once food leaves the stomach, it reaches the duodenum, where a different set of enzymes goes to work. These enzymes are produced by the pancreas and the liver, on the one hand, and by the intestine itself, on the other. Together, they split up the food into usable microscopic fragments. The most important of these enzymes are the lipase, the amylase, and the peptidase. They are responsible for splitting the food into individual molecules, breaking down proteins, and transforming carbohydrates into smaller molecules, such as glucose, fructose, and galactose. With the help of enzymes, the proteins contained in our food are split into their individual components, the amino acids.

There are a total of 20 amino acids, eight of which are classified as "essential," meaning necessary for normal health and growth. The eight essential amino acids are leucine, isoleucine, lysine, phenylalanine, methionine, threonine, tryptophan, and valine. Whereas carbohydrates supply energy to the body, the amino acids in proteins fulfill a number of different tasks. Some are important for muscles and connective tissue, others for nerves and the brain. Still others influence our mental well-being and have

Tip

If you have a sensitive stomach, avoid fried foods and foods with a grilled-cheese topping, because the digestive enzymes take a long time breaking down these foods.

The intestine can only absorb and utilize nutrients with the help of digestive enzymes.

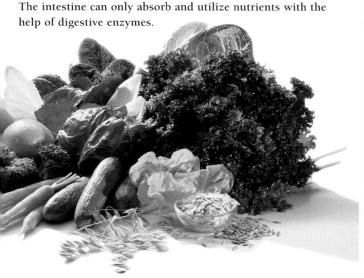

15

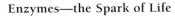

a direct relationship to our susceptibility to stress. It isn't easy for enzymes to break down the amino acids in foods, because they are made up of complex chains. The digestive enzymes in the stomach and the small intestine first need to crack the links between the individual chains.

How Fat Is Dissolved

Fats and oils do not dissolve in water; instead, they form little droplets. These droplets make it difficult for the enzymes that break down fat to attack. In order to circumvent this, the bile produced by the liver contains bile acids that, just like dishwashing detergent, dissolve the fatty droplets. Only then can the enzymes (produced by the pancreas) break down fats and oils into their individual components.

Once all nutrients have been broken down, different enzymes are responsible for transporting them through the wall of the intestine into the blood and on to the cells waiting in the body. Enzymes also transport essential vitamins and minerals from the intestine into the blood. The unusable remains of the food continue to the large intestine, where, again, enzymes trigger the process of fermentation necessary for eventual excretion.

Safeguards in the Enzyme World

As there are thousands of different enzymes working in the body, the question is, how does each individual enzyme know where to go? For instance, is it possible for an enzyme that is supposed to supply oxygen to mistakenly end up with those enzymes intended to break down food? This would cause considerable damage, because the enzyme wouldn't know anything about breaking down food. To prevent such a mistake from taking place, the body has established a protection mechanism. Scientists call this mechanism "substrate specificity," which means that a specific enzyme will only break down the substance that it is intended to break down.

Like a Key in a Lock

Each enzyme is assigned a specific place of action and will reach that place. If an enzyme appears at the wrong place,

Tip
You can encourage enzyme production in your stomach and intestine by chewing your food well and cooking with lots of aromatic herbs and spices. If your body produces sufficient amounts of digestive enzymes, then you won't suffer from indigestion and your intestines will be able to utilize the nutrients in the food fully.

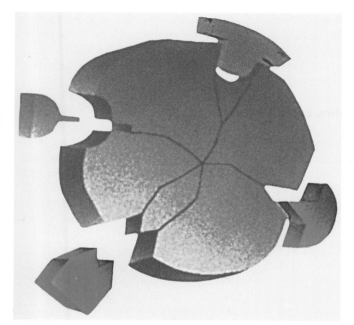

Just as a key turns only in the lock for which it is intended, the shape of an enzyme determines where it will go to work.

To understand how enzymes work where they are supposed to, it may help to picture the human body as a city. The houses in this city represent the substrates, and the inhabitants of the houses stand for the enzymes. Every house (substrate) has a lock on its door, and every inhabitant (enzyme) has the key to only his or her door. The inhabitants will not be able to gain access to any other house but their own.

it won't cause any damage, because it will not be able to gain entry. Just as a key only fits the keyhole it is cut for, an enzyme only belongs to one substance (substrate)—for all other substrates, the door remains locked. Therefore, an enzyme that breaks down fatty acids cannot interfere with the breakdown of sugars or proteins.

Fatal Errors

Despite all safeguards, accidents do happen when enzymes are at work. Some years back, a few cost-conscious vintners in Europe tried to make their harvest stretch further by adding antifreeze to the juice of the grapes. The seemingly clever vintners were counting on the effects of an enzyme called alcohol dehydrogenase (probably without ever having heard of it).

As a rule, this enzyme breaks down ethyl alcohol, which

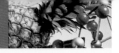

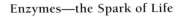

is contained in alcoholic drinks like beer and wine. Yet it also breaks down ethylene glycol, the main ingredient of antifreeze, because the enzyme mistakes it for ethyl alcohol. What the vintners didn't know is that antifreeze will only become dangerous for humans as a result of this enzyme activity, as it enables the toxins released in the breakdown process to be transported to the kidneys. The only remedy in this case is to get completely and utterly drunk, because if the prodigal enzyme is fed real ethyl alcohol, it loses interest in the "substitute drug," which will then be flushed out of the body without causing any harm. The vintners were not aware of the rare possibility that errors like these could occur. The enzymes were their downfall, and unfortunately a number of consumers were harmed as a result.

If the body has to make do with a reduced intake of nutrients during a weight-loss diet, the enzymes in the body will automatically eat into the existing reserves. Unfortunately, this exerts a great strain on the heart, where significant amounts of protein are stored. For this reason, no one should fast or eat a low-calorie, low-protein diet over a long duration without being closely monitored by a doctor.

Enzymes Work If and When Needed

Enzymes are programmed to take breaks if the amount of work done, for the time being, ensures that the body will function normally. If, for instance, enough carbohydrates have been converted into glucose to have some energy in reserve, enzyme activity will come to a halt. It will start again, however, before the reserves are depleted, so that there will never be a shortage of supplies in the body.

Unfortunately, it is here that people today often interfere and upset the routine by their unhealthy eating habits. If you eat a one-sided diet—for example, by ingesting large amounts of fat—the enzymes that specialize in breaking down carbohydrates will remain idle. Almost no enzymes will work fast enough if you don't consume a sufficient amount of vitamins and minerals. As far as the surplus is concerned, enzymes utilize the amounts that are needed at the time and store the remainder, regardless of whether it is fat, protein, or carbohydrates. This is where any extra padding comes from that we may discover on our buttocks, stomachs, and thighs.

Proenzymes on Call

Millions of enzymes roam through the body in the blood without being active. In this passive state, they are called proenzymes and have a structure that differs from that of active enzymes. Amino acids break up the protein chain of the enzyme in a specific place, thus rendering it incapable of doing any work. If it is needed, however, another enzyme will remove the amino acids, leaving a fully functioning enzyme ready to do the work for which it was intended. This safeguard, for example, prevents enzymes from digesting the stomach should there be no food in it. On the one hand, the stomach's natural lining protects it from attacks, and, on the other, the enzyme pepsin will remain in its proenzyme form, pepsinogen, until it is activated by the gastric acid. With the arrival of food—that is, with work—gastric acid springs into action.

One problem occurs, however: A once-activated enzyme can no longer be reconverted into its passive state. But when all food has been broken down and utilized, the enzymes will need to take a break. The body produces inhibitors for this purpose that block the center of the enzyme.

How Enzymes React to Heat

Enzyme activity depends on body temperature. The best results are achieved at 96.8 degrees Fahrenheit (36 degrees Celsius). Enzyme productivity decreases at lower temperatures, and enzymes go into overdrive in the case of a fever. Higher temperatures generally encourage enzyme activity, resulting in a boost for the metabolism. This happens for a good reason, because now the body will activate all possible resources to fight an illness. A fever is therefore not the result of harmful bacteria or viruses invading the body; it is instead the immune system's response to these pathogens.

Initially, a fever is a healthy reaction by the body to an illness, as it indicates that the immune system is active. This is linked to enzymes in the body's defenses, because a raised temperature increases enzyme activity. It is therefore not advisable to suppress a slight fever immediately with medication. However, if the fever rises a great deal within a short period of time, it puts a strain on the already weakened body, and thus the temperature should be lowered.

19

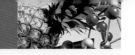

Strengthening the Body's Defenses

We are not able to cover in this book the innumerable tasks performed by the individual enzymes. Enzymes play a part in everything that takes place within the body, from the clotting of blood to the functioning of the nervous system, the heart, the liver, and the kidneys. Here, our focus is specifically those areas where enzymes are of particular significance to our health, such as the immune system. Our bodies' defenses are essential to our vitality. The strength of our defenses determines whether we will catch an infection or not, how hard an illness will hit us, and how quickly we will recuperate. Even the way we handle everyday stress depends largely on how well our bodies' defenses work.

> Numerous enzymes are necessary to break down nicotine and alcohol. If you avoid these poisons, your body will have more enzymes available to fight bacteria and viruses.

The Body's Defensive Strategy

Like a general, the defenses of the human body strive to prevent the enemy from breaking through the lines. The enemy appears in the form of viruses, bacteria, fungi, and many other germs that can cause considerable damage to the body. A poorly armed attacker will fail at the first obstacle, the skin, because its acid environment presents an effective deterrent. In addition to the skin, the enemy may try to enter through one of the orifices of the body.

Enzymes at the Front

The attack through the mouth and the nose is no less tricky. Both have a protective lining that is home to a particularly aggressive enzyme called lysozyme. This enzyme is capable of dissolving adversaries completely. Other enemies hide in food; however, they will usually advance no further than the stomach, where they will fall victim to gastric acid. If an enemy is well camouflaged or faced with weakened defenses, it may advance as far as the blood supply. At this point, the immune system resorts to heavier weapons: the killer cells and the macrophages. Both are

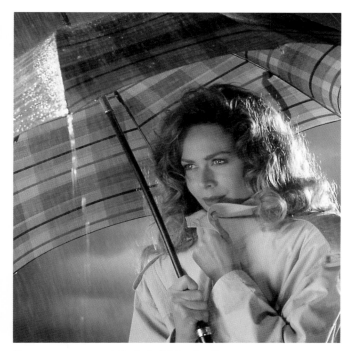

Enzymes are especially helpful in the flu season.

formed in the white blood cells. The latter, which are tissue
cells, simply consume the intruders, whereas the killer cells
attack again and again until the enemy is destroyed.

Spies on the Battlefield

Should a Trojan horse—that is, a particularly well camouflaged enemy—enter the body, then antibodies, the spies in
the body's defense lines, come into action. They chase the
enemy mercilessly and with their presence alert the other
defense mechanisms, especially the macrophages. The antibodies stick to the intruder like glue until it is destroyed.

This combination of antibodies and attackers is called
an immune complex. By sending out signals, antibodies
can call on another special unit for help: the complementary system. This special unit of the body intervenes when-

21

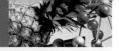

ever the macrophages are unable to reach the attacker. Such is the case when the immune complex has already settled down in the body's tissue, because the macrophages can only destroy intruders that swim around freely in the blood. The complementary system, however, destroys the surrounding tissue as well.

When Enzymes Are Involved

Enzymes are highly active in this kind of battle. Research is far from exhaustive with regard to what takes place in the body when it fights an infection, and the many roles of enzymes, in particular, are still unclear. It is certain, however, that they encourage the macrophages to do the best they can. Try to picture an enzyme whipping the macrophage into shape and causing it to consume intruders up to 10 times faster than it had.

Enzyme activity can be measured in the blood, as can the increased activity of the macrophages. Researchers took blood from a test person and examined the activities of both enzymes and macrophages. They then gave the person an enzyme preparation, drew another blood sample, and checked again. The result was that the enzymes had already sent the macrophages into overdrive. In record time, they destroyed the foreign substances that had been given to the test person. This test proves that taking an enzyme preparation does actually improve the body's defenses.

Other enzymes already active in the skin perform perhaps more menial services by quickly removing the remains of the slain enemy, thus preventing immune complexes from forming.

When Immune Complexes Turn Dangerous

Modern science is mainly interested in those protein-splitting enzymes that are capable of removing immune complexes from the tissue and redirecting them into the bloodstream. There, they will be destroyed by the macrophages before they are able to harm the body. In order to understand how damaging immune complexes can be, we should recall that initially they are produced

Enzyme therapy can provide quick assistance in the case of acute illnesses. If the body's defenses are generally weakened, however, it may take weeks or even months for enzyme treatment to take effect.

with the best of intentions. As we have mentioned, antibodies latch onto an enemy, thus signaling to the macrophages and the complementary system that here is an enemy waiting to be destroyed. However, the macrophages can only harm the immune complexes if they swim around freely in the bloodstream.

Unfortunately, immune complexes sometimes attach themselves to tissue, leaving the macrophages without a chance. Only the complementary system can help, but it sometimes becomes overzealous. It doesn't just destroy the enemy attached to the antibody—it can also destroy the surrounding tissue and even entire organs. This means that the complementary system can no longer distinguish between friend or foe and unintentionally causes considerable damage.

Enzymes vs. Immune Complexes

Depending on where in the tissue an immune complex has attached itself, it can cause severe damage to the skin, the intestine, the joints, the lungs, or the kidneys. If one's own immune system causes damage to the body, this is referred to by doctors as an autoimmune disorder. Examples of such a disorder are chronic polyarthritis, which affects two or more joints, and multiple sclerosis, which affects the nervous system.

The pharmaceutical industry is busy working on the development of enzyme preparations that could tackle the cause of an autoimmune disorder—namely, the immune complexes that have attached themselves to the tissue. If enzyme preparations were successful in separating all these immune complexes from their tissue, many dangerous diseases would finally be conquered.

Immune complexes have a part in autoimmune disorders such as rheumatism and multiple sclerosis.

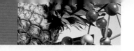

Coenzymes—the Enzymes' Little Helpers

Most enzymes can't do their work alone—they need the support of other biological substances called coenzymes. Some support the enzyme directly, working together with it. In this way, iron improves the absorption of oxygen. Others aren't useful to the enzyme in their original form, but are needed to make up yet further substances that the enzyme requires.

Sources of Coenzymes

The term "coenzymes" refers to those substances that work directly in conjunction with an enzyme and those that help to build other substances. The most important coenzymes are the B vitamins, vitamin C, minerals, and trace elements. Unlike enzymes, coenzymes are not produced in the body (in sufficient amounts), but they have to be taken daily through the food in our diet. If we don't consume a sufficient amount of coenzymes, enzyme activity in our bodies will be impaired.

Irreplaceable: The B Vitamins

B vitamins work closely with numerous enzymes that play an important role in supplying the body with oxygen and in forming individual cells. In order to provide vitality and energy, cells need nutrients and oxygen. Only then can they grow and divide again and again.

- **Niacin** (vitamin B3) is required by enzymes to fulfill important tasks in cell metabolism. So that the cell enzymes can use niacin, it undergoes a slight biochemical change and is converted into what scientists call NAD or NADP (one has a slightly different structure from the other). Niacin is contained in lean meats, poultry, fish, and mushrooms.
- **Pantothenic acid** (vitamin B5) is required by the enzymes that convert food into energy and lay down stores for emergencies. This vitamin is contained in

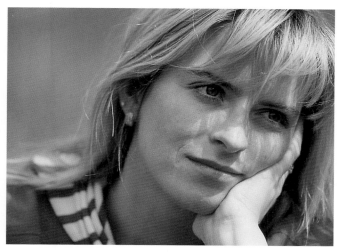

A coenzyme deficiency can be the cause of listlessness and a lack of concentration.

Studies have shown that weight-loss diets often lead to a B-vitamin deficiency, which in turn decreases enzyme metabolism.

whole-grain products, sweetbreads, wheat bran, and green vegetables.

- **Vitamin B6** (pyridoxine) is also one of the metabolic vitamins, but it has a special function with regard to enzymes. It mainly assists those enzymes that work on the amino acids that the body needs for the formation of essential protein molecules. Whole-wheat products, avocados, beans, bananas, nuts, yeast, wheat germ, and liver are particularly rich in vitamin B6.
- **Biotin** is also considered a B vitamin. It helps the enzymes break down carbohydrates so that the body can utilize the energy they provide. Biotin is contained in liver, egg yolks, oats, soybeans, rice, and yeast.
- **Folic acid,** another B vitamin, assists the enzyme that contributes to the formation of hemoglobin. It also plays a part in the correct formation of the genetic code. Folic acid is contained in cabbage, carrots, spinach, beans, and whole-grain products.

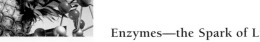

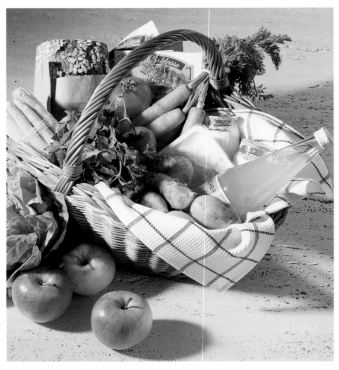

Coenzymes from the B-vitamin group are often sadly lacking on our dinner tables. Young women, in particular, don't seem to get sufficient amounts of these vital coenzymes. A varied diet is all that is needed to remedy the problem.

The vitamins and minerals contained in our food are counted among the coenzymes without which many enzymes couldn't function.

B Vitamins Especially Good for the Nervous System

- **Vitamin B1** (thiamin) is of significance for enzyme activity in the nervous system, especially for the error-free transmission of stimuli that is controlled by the brain. A thiamin deficiency and the lack of related enzyme activity can result in irritability, aggressiveness, listlessness, despondency, insomnia, or loss of appetite. Vitamin B1 is found in pork, legumes, whole-grain products, vegetables, wheat germ, potatoes, yeast, nuts, seeds, and liver.
- **Vitamin B2** (riboflavin) assists numerous enzymes responsible for the metabolism of proteins, fats, and car-

bohydrates. It also supports the enzymes that regulate nervous activity. If these enzymes cannot function properly due to a lack of vitamin B2, depression or a lack of concentration may result. Vitamin B2 is found in sweetbreads, dairy products, whole-grain products, and fish. It is one of the coenzymes that undergo some restructuring in the body; the resultant coenzyme is known by the abbreviation FAD.

- **Vitamin B12** (cobalamin) supports the enzymes in the nervous system and those that are responsible for the formation of red blood cells. It can be found in sweetbreads, meat, fish, and eggs.

Q10—a Fountain of Youth?

Q10, or ubiquinone, achieved some fame a few years back. Hardly anyone had heard of Q10 until certain advertising campaigns started claiming it was the key to eternal youth. The coenzyme Q10 ranks foremost among the substances necessary to sustain life, as it plays a part in cell respiration, which in turn is the prerequisite for cell growth and cell division. Its other task is to bind free radicals, which are dangerous molecular fragments that can cause severe damage to cells and can even cause cancer. Q10 is found in all foods, but it is also produced by the body itself.

The human body produces the coenzyme Q10 itself. Large amounts of it are also contained in meat, fish, and many other foods.

Yet contrary to what some advertisers have said, we haven't discovered the fountain of youth with Q10. It is true that the Q10 content in cells decreases steadily with age, but this is also the case with other biological substances; for this reason, Q10 cannot be regarded as the sole cause of aging.

Coenzymes from Mother Earth

Over the past few years, science has focused more and more on minerals and trace elements. Doctors have discovered mineral and trace element deficiencies in many patients. There are two main reasons for these deficiencies: Excessively fertilized soil is being increasingly depleted of nutrients, and our diets are consisting of more low-nutrient fast foods and fewer fresh foods.

Mineral deficiencies can bring about the symptoms of

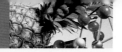

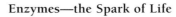

various illnesses, but our main interest in this book is the fact that a lack of minerals immobilizes numerous enzymes. Many enzymes depend on minerals to do their work. Trace elements are also minerals, but the body needs only very small quantities of them.

Minerals Supply Energy

- **Potassium** is the substance for which athletes and people who do hard physical labor have the greatest need, because the body loses it through perspiration. A potassium deficiency is hardly ever caused by a poor diet—it is nearly always the result of increased excretion, such as through perspiration. Potassium is mainly required for the proper functioning of the muscles in our bodies, and a lack of potassium could even result in heart problems. One of the most important metabolic enzymes, pyruvate kinase, depends on potassium to a large extent.

  If you demand maximum performance of your body, you should consume 2 to 3 quarts, or liters, of fluids per day. Fruit and vegetable juices are best, whereas care should be taken with mineral water, because not all brands contain a sufficient amount of potassium. Make sure you read the label on the bottle. Potassium can also be found in mushrooms, wheat bran, apricots, bananas, and vegetables.

- **Sodium** is one of the basic minerals in the human body. Sodium deficiencies are practically unheard of, as sodium is contained in normal cooking salt and mineral water. There is a risk, however, of excessive sodium intake. Sodium supports muscle function and tissue tension, the so-called osmotic pressure of the body fluids. One enzyme, in particular, depends on sodium: ATPase, which supplies the cells with energy so that they can function properly.

- **Magnesium** stimulates a number of metabolic enzymes—without it as a catalyst, they would remain inactive. Magnesium is indispensable especially in regard to cell metabolism. Its protective properties for nerves and muscles have been known for a long time now. Magnesium works closely with all enzymes that are

Tip

The body often loses large amounts of potassium and other minerals after severe bouts of diarrhea or as a result of long-term use of laxatives. It is important that you compensate for these losses quickly by eating plenty of vegetables and drinking mineral water.

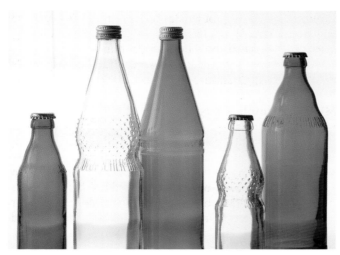

Various brands of mineral water differ in their mineral content.

responsible for heart and circulatory activity. The combination of magnesium with its numerous enzymes helps us cope better with everyday stresses and strains, and suffer less from stress-related illnesses. It also prevents heart problems. Dairy products, whole-grain products, fruit, vegetables, liver, and fish are all good sources of magnesium.

Trace Elements Help Maintain Youthful Vigor

- **Iron** is essential for the formation of hemoglobin, the coloring matter of red blood cells. Hemoglobin moves oxygen in the blood from the lungs to the tissues, which require oxygen to maintain the basic life functions. Numerous enzymes play a part in supplying the body's cells with oxygen. None of these enzymes would function without iron, and cells would age and cease to function sooner. Liver, lean meat, whole-grain products, vegetables, and legumes are all good sources of iron.
- **Copper** is needed by iron, because it wouldn't be able to enter the red blood cells without it. Copper also forms part of the cells of the immune system, and it sup-

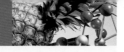

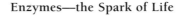

ports an important analgesic and anti-inflammatory enzyme called SOD. This is why copper is used in the treatment of many rheumatic disorders. Copper can mainly be found in nuts, fish, meat, leafy green vegetables, and legumes.

- **Zinc** is part of no less than 160 enzymes that are active in our cells, the immune system, and our metabolism. Zinc spurs those enzymes into action that are responsible for beautiful skin. They improve blood circulation and ensure that toxins leave the system quickly and that the skin receives an optimal supply of nutrients. You can admire the results daily in the mirror: Your skin will stay smooth, wrinkle-free, rosy, and young longer. Seafood, eggs, organ meats, wheat germ, and soybeans contain large amounts of zinc.

- **Manganese** is needed by the enzymes in connective tissue to form fibers that ensure that the tissue will be firm yet elastic. Manganese also assists the biotin enzyme, which is important for the metabolism of carbohydrates. Wheat bran, oats, hazelnuts, and whole-grain products are good sources of manganese.

- **Selenium** protects cells from viral infections and helps to prevent cancer and joint problems. It is also part of an important detoxifying enzyme (glutathione peroxidase) that breaks down the damaging free radicals. As if this weren't enough, selenium also renders heavy metals such as mercury, lead, and cadmium harmless by firmly bonding with them. Because the soil contains less and less selenium, many plants increasingly contain less of it as well. In addition to nuts, whole grains are still a good plant-based source of selenium. However, sweetbreads and fish contain much higher amounts.

Tip

Acid rain has resulted in grains and bakery products containing less and less selenium. However, if you are frequently exposed to heavy metals or exhaust fumes, you will need large amounts of selenium to detoxify your body. Selenium supplements will quickly remedy any deficiency.

Enzyme Therapy— Pineapple or Pills?

Sometimes the body's enzymes need a gentle prodding from the outside. And then the question arises: Do I supplement my enzyme stocks with pills and other medications, or can I just eat foods that are rich in enzymes?

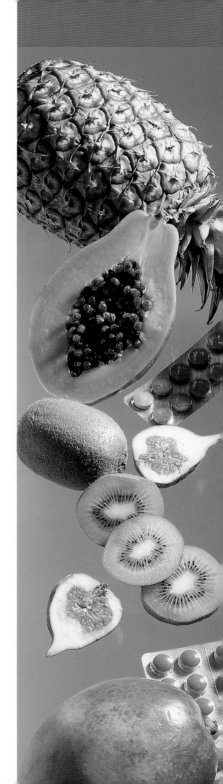

When There Is an Enzyme Deficiency

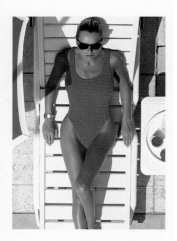

Excessive sunbathing not only damages your skin; overexposure to ultraviolet rays can also cause genetic defects. Usually, they remain without consequences, but if they cause an enzyme to be produced improperly, serious metabolic disorders may be the result.

By and large, enzymes are very reliable. The body usually produces them in sufficient amounts and normally they function effectively. We say normally, because there are a number of factors that can block enzyme activity, such as genetic disorders, a poor diet, environmental toxins, and illnesses. Fortunately, major enzyme deficiencies are fairly rare, but when they occur, they have far-reaching consequences.

Malfunctioning Cells

A genetic error in the setup of a cell can, for example, result in the program for the production of an enzyme not functioning properly or in the program not existing at all. Research has pinpointed several causes for these changes in the genetic structure: X rays, radioactive radiation, ultraviolet radiation, chemicals, certain infectious diseases, and others. Modern science cannot yet prevent the causes of such defects, but this is an area that could benefit from gene technology sometime in the future.

At the present time, medicine can only diagnose which enzyme is lacking. Nevertheless, there are no substitutes for missing enzymes, which means that the person concerned must avoid all foods that his or her body is unable to metabolize because of the missing enzyme.

Coenzyme Deficiencies

Vitamins, minerals, and trace elements are all coenzymes. If your body does not receive sufficient amounts of these coenzymes from your diet, then the enzymes will not be able to function properly.

Yet fresh, high-quality foods alone will not do the trick, because coenzymes are highly sensitive and have dangerous enemies. To ensure that your food actually contains the vitamins and other nutrients that your body requires, it has to be handled carefully.

Treating Coenzymes Gently

- Coenzymes aren't very fond of long journeys around the world and extended stays in your storage cupboard or refrigerator. After only three days, many foods lose up to 60 percent of their vitamins. Even if food is refrigerated, it loses up to 20 percent of its vitamin C after three days. Therefore, choose fresh, seasonal foods that are produced locally.
- Overcooking destroys the sensitive coenzymes. So, go easy on your food when you prepare a meal—who says that vegetables shouldn't be crunchy?
- All B vitamins, vitamin C, and all minerals are water-soluble, which means they may be lost if foods are washed too vigorously or boiled in water. Vegetables containing B vitamins and vitamin C should always be washed first and then chopped, sliced, etc.
- Steam your vegetables, or use just a little water for cooking. This way, an average of 70 to 80 percent of the water-soluble coenzymes will remain in the vegetables. If vegetables are boiled in water, about half of the vitamins are usually lost.
- If your children are late for dinner, don't keep it warm, because most vitamins won't survive. Let the food cool down, and reheat it only when everybody is seated around the table.
- Blanch vegetables shortly before freezing them, because they often contain enzymes that damage vitamins and continue to work even in the freezer. A brief spell in hot water will destroy them, however.
- Milk contains large amounts of the coenzyme vitamin B2, which, unfortunately, is very sensitive to light. The neon lights of the cooling counters are like poison to these important nutrients. Therefore, choose milk cartons, which protect the vitamins.

Tip
Choose organic produce, because it is grown in soil that has not been excessively fertilized. Fruit and vegetables can therefore absorb sufficient amounts of minerals.

Weight-Loss Diets

A one-sided diet will always cause a deficiency of certain vitamins and minerals. It disturbs the enzyme balance, because it jeopardizes the supply of coenzymes. This doesn't always remain without consequences—after all, enzymes strengthen the body's defenses. If the body lacks enzymes, it will not be able to cope with illnesses as well as usual.

Furthermore, most people don't know that enzymes are responsible for rapid weight gain after a strict diet. The human body is designed to store energy for emergencies. Any fat and sugar that it doesn't need immediately are converted and deposited in stores. But if you want to lose weight, you would like to see those stores disappear. By keeping to a diet, the body believes an emergency situation has arisen and it is allowed to use its emergency rations. This produces the desired result: You lose those extra pounds. But alas, once the diet is over and you give in to your cravings for cakes and burgers, this sends the enzymes into overdrive. Never again will they allow such an emergency to occur, and so they convert every last bit of food to restock the empty stores. Thus, the vicious cycle of weight loss and weight gain begins. You will gain weight more quickly after a diet, thanks to those diligent enzymes.

Tip
Vitamin and mineral supplements can compensate for a lack of coenzymes. Choose multivitamin and mineral preparations, and carefully adhere to the instructions for dosage. Occasionally, taking too much can be harmful (for example, with vitamins A and D).

Medications, Alcohol, and Cigarettes
Laxatives, antibiotics, a number of painkillers, and medicines for rheumatism all prevent the absorption of the B vitamins. Antibiotics also cause an increased need for vitamins A, C, and E, and laxatives also pose a threat to the body's mineral balance. By far the most dangerous vitamin thieves are cigarettes (vitamin C), alcohol (vitamin A and all B vitamins), and stress. Constant stress severely depletes the B vitamins, which are vital for enzyme activity. Emotional strain damages the entire body and also encourages the formation of the dangerous free radicals. If you can't escape stress, it is advisable to take supplements containing all the important B vitamins, vitamin E, beta-carotene, selenium, and magnesium.

Environmental Poisons Kill Enzymes
Environmental poisons are a relatively new source of danger to our health. Apart from the physical damage they can cause, environmental poisons also obstruct enzyme activity. They act as inhibitors, blocking vital enzymes, and this can

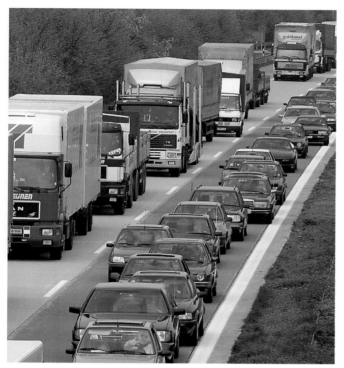

It is almost impossible to avoid environmental poisons. However, usually the body activates enzymes that break down toxins.

The body possesses enzymes that break down environmental toxins. You can support these enzymes by eating foods that are rich in selenium. Good sources of selenium are whole grains (there are special breads with a high selenium content), fish, and nuts.

result in serious illness. The most dangerous environmental poisons are carbon monoxide, mercury, lead, cadmium, copper compounds, and cyanide. Truck drivers, factory workers, and people who live in highly polluted areas should monitor their health carefully. If symptoms of an illness appear, the cause may well be an enzyme deficiency.

Aging Slows Down Enzyme Production

Enzymes are biocatalysts. They trigger or accelerate reactions in the body. With increasing age, many bodily functions slow down. This is not surprising, as all the previously mentioned factors, such as one-sided diets,

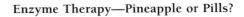

How to Avoid Enzyme Killers

- If your plumbing consists of old copper pipes, run your faucet for a couple of minutes each morning before you use the water to make tea or coffee.
- Don't buy fruit or vegetables from a stall next to a busy street, because the pollutants from the exhaust fumes will settle on the produce.
- Fruit and vegetables with a smooth surface should not merely be washed but also rubbed down with a sponge, as this is the best way to remove the toxins that cling to the surface.
- Cadmium is found particularly in kidneys. It would therefore be best to avoid eating kidneys of any kind very often.

With increasing age, the pancreas produces only 60 percent of the enzymes it used to produce in younger years. In many older people, this can cause digestive problems.

medications, and environmental poisons, influence the body's enzyme balance over time, leaving their marks. Digestive problems are a typical example of the consequences enzyme deficiencies can have. Furthermore, enzymes age and show signs of wear and tear. Their strength is reduced with growing pressure, and the production of new enzymes takes longer and longer. Depending on your individual circumstances, this process can start when you are in your thirties, and most people in their forties will suffer from certain enzyme deficiencies.

Does a Special Enzyme Diet Work?

Numerous foods not only contain coenzymes (vitamins, minerals, and trace elements) but enzymes as well. A good combination, one would think, but it's far from it! The natural enzymes found in foods are so sensitive that it is almost impossible to cover increased enzyme requirements through our diet.

Which Foods Contain Enzymes?

In general, enzymes can be found in all raw foods, but especially in fruit and vegetables. Three of the most important enzymes from our diet are contained in tropical fruit.

- Pineapple contains bromelain, an enzyme that splits up proteins and assists with the removal of toxins and waste products from the body. Because of the latter, it plays an important role in weight-loss diets.

Pineapple and papaya are considered slimming foods, because they contain enzymes. However, their enzymes break down proteins and are entirely unsuitable for dissolving fat stores.

Tip
The enzymes in tropical fruit are very unpopular in the kitchen, because they split up proteins. This is why cottage cheese mixed with pieces of kiwi fruit will taste bitter after a while. Gelatin will never become solid when pineapple is around, because it contains proteins that cannot withstand the enzymes in the pineapple. To reduce the effect of the enzymes, briefly blanch the fruit with boiling water.

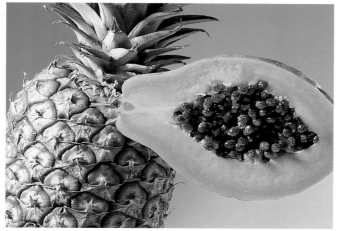

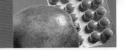

- Papain is the enzyme contained in papaya. It can break down 35 times its own volume in animal proteins and make it available for the body to use—it's a true power source!
- Kiwifruit also contains a protein-splitting enzyme called actinidine. This causes the proteins in dairy products to turn bitter.

Enzyme Sensitivity

Enzymes need to be treated with even greater care than vitamins. They react badly to changes in temperature; in fact, temperatures above 104 degrees Fahrenheit (40 degrees Celsius) destroy them completely, which means they must not be cooked. They can, however, cope with freezing, as this merely causes them to stop working temporarily. As soon as temperatures become more enzyme-friendly, they resume their work.

Enzymes suffer most from long storage times, whether in markets or storage cupboards or owing to a long journey from their country of origin—they just don't survive. For the enzymes to be effective, the foods in which they are found have to be eaten fresh. Here lies the problem with fruit such as pineapple and papaya that may have to be flown in from far away—by the time they are eaten, they have lost a lot of their power.

Enzymes Killed in the Stomach

Many enzymes have already been lost by the time we eat a piece of fruit, and as if this weren't enough, our bodies destroy a large portion of the remaining enzymes. The food in the stomach comes under attack from hydrochloric acid, which destroys germs and breaks down all protein molecules. This is the source of the problem, as enzymes are protein molecules and therefore have little chance of surviving the onslaught of the gastric acid. The living conditions for enzymes improve once they reach the intestine. From there, they travel through the intestinal wall into the bloodstream and the lymphatic fluid. However, natural enzymes from our diet never make it that far.

Enzymes from the Pharmacy

Two thousand years ago, open wounds were treated by applying fresh figs, as we can glean from the Bible. Around 1900, the first medical trials took place in which attempts at healing were made by injecting plant- and animal-based enzymes. Up to the mid-twentieth century, only inborn enzyme defects were treated. The enzyme preparations we can purchase today from pharmacies and health food stores (and administer ourselves) have only been available since the 1960s.

Ask for enzyme preparations that are manufactured in such a way that gastric acid cannot destroy them.

"And Isaiah said, Take a lump of figs. And they took it and laid it on the boil, and he recovered." —Old Testament, Book of Kings

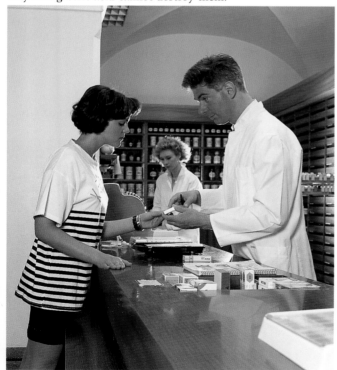

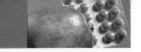

Treatment for the Whole System

Using enzymes to treat several different complaints is called "systemic enzyme therapy" by the experts. "Systemic," here, means that the enzymes are distributed in the body via the bloodstream. Enzyme therapy can loosely be regarded as a natural treatment, because it stimulates the self-healing powers of the body in a natural manner.

Many enzyme preparations contain animal-based enzymes (pancreatin, trypsin, and chymotrypsin) as well as plant-based enzymes (bromelain, which is obtained from the stalk of the pineapple, and papain, procured from the leaves and the unripe fruit of the papaya tree). Bromelain and papain are both capable of reducing swelling. They break down large protein molecules in the tissue and remove them. This lessens the swelling and alleviates the pressure on the nerves, which in turn means less pain. Animal-based enzymes dissolve solid blood clots and flush the fragments away with the blood. Therefore, if you have a tooth extracted, you will not have to suffer from a swollen, bruised cheek for very long.

Any worries that animal-based enzymes could stem from BSE-infected cattle (cattle with "mad cow disease") are unfounded. Only chymotrypsin is obtained from cows, and this is imported from countries where no cases of BSE have been reported.

Most enzyme pills contain a mix of animal- and plant-based enzymes. The advantage of this is that a single enzyme preparation is able to treat a number of ailments.

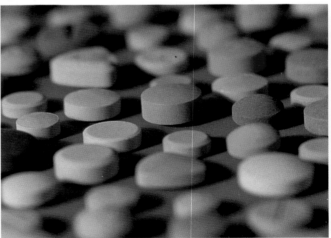

The Most Important Enzymes and Their Uses

Enzyme Range of Application

Bromelain	Helps to combat chronic inflammations and autoimmune diseases, supports the treatment of vein complaints and thrombosis, helps to prevent sports injuries, and assists in the preparation for surgery
Chymotrypsin	Useful in treating chronic inflammations and immune complex illnesses (also see trypsin)
Papain	Helps treat immune complex illnesses, injuries, swelling, and chronic inflammations
Pepsin	Helps alleviate digestive trouble and a lack of appetite
Trypsin	Helps to alleviate vein complaints and thrombosis and to prevent cancer and arteriosclerosis

Tip
Enzyme therapy can often cause the color, shape, or smell of one's stools to change. With very high dosages, feelings of fullness and flatulence have been reported occasionally. These reactions can be avoided, however, if the tablets are taken at intervals spaced out throughout the day. Trials have shown that even a daily dosage of 100 tablets has no ill effects on the patient.

Effective without Side Effects

Even if enzymes are taken in high doses over a long period of time—for example, six months—they do not usually have any side effects. Very rarely do allergic reactions occur, and, when they do, they disappear without further consequences once the enzyme therapy has been discontinued.

Initially, one of the problems systemic enzyme therapy posed was to find a way to allow the enzymes to reach the intestine despite the aggressive gastric acid. As discussed previously, this is not possible with the enzymes that are contained in our food. But the pharmaceutical industry came up with a solution: Enzyme tablets were given a coating that could not be dissolved immediately, even by the

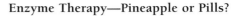

aggressive gastric acid, granting the tablets time to reach the intestine before releasing the enzymes.

The fairly high dosages that the patient has to take (manufacturers generally recommend four tablets three times a day) cannot be altered. Research over the years has shown that it is necessary to supply as many enzymes as possible to their place of work. Consider the following:

1. One tablet can only accommodate a limited amount of enzymes, and larger tablets are more difficult to swallow.
2. Some of the sensitive enzymes are destroyed by acids on their journey through the body—this is unavoidable.
3. At some point, however, these acids will be "sated" and the remaining enzymes can then travel on to their destinations without any further obstacles.

Successful Self-Treatment

Because you don't have to worry about side effects from enzyme preparations, they can be wholeheartedly recommended for the self-treatment of many ailments. For some,

For many disorders and chronic diseases, self-treatment is perfectly acceptable once a diagnosis has been established. If you aren't sure about the cause of your symptoms, consult your physician.

How to Take Enzymes

If you are using enzyme preparations, it is recommended to take higher doses rather than lower doses. In the case of an acute illness, start with a high dosage and then phase the medication out slowly. Enzyme therapy can be continued over a long period of time without any risk.

In some cases, it is possible to inject enzymes, but this should only be done with proper medical supervision. Usually, enzymes are taken in the form of tablets; but in the case of severe illnesses (cancer, for instance), when nausea and so forth make taking medication orally difficult, enzymes can be administered rectally by means of an enema. This method allows a surprisingly large amount of enzymes to be absorbed. It is interesting to note that in all enzyme preparations the same enzymes are effective. A multienzyme preparation will therefore help you to treat a number of ailments.

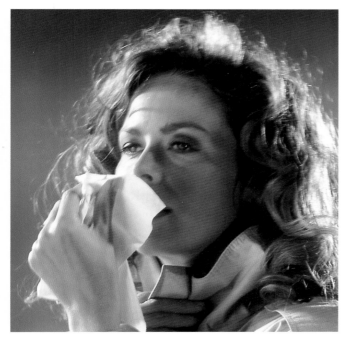

A combination of conventional medications and enzyme preparations has proven useful in the treatment of nasal sinus infections.

Do not discontinue any medication your doctor has prescribed without consulting him or her first, even if you feel much improved as a result of enzyme therapy.

they can be the sole treatment; for others, they can be used to support conventional therapeutic measures.

Enzymes Can Act as "Tugboats"

Enzyme preparations have displayed an optimizing effect when taken in conjunction with certain conventional medicines such as antibiotics and cytostatics (used in the treatment of malignant tumors). Scientists have observed repeatedly that there was an increased concentration of the medication in the affected tissue when enzyme preparations were taken simultaneously. This is particularly helpful for patients who need to take strong medication over a long period of time. In addition, with illnesses where the medication can only reach its destination with difficulty (as

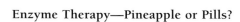

with prostate complaints or sinus infections), enzymes can act as "tugboats" that take the required medicine to its destination. This method has been utilized for some time in ointments that are applied to wounds.

Later on, you will find an overview of some of the illnesses that respond well to enzyme therapy. The table below lists those complaints that you can treat with enzymes yourself.

When Enzymes Are Useful

As a preventive measure for:
- An increased risk of injury (for instance, in the case of athletes)
- Vein complaints and arteriosclerosis
- Age-related complaints

In the treatment of:
- Joint diseases
- Virus infections
- Injuries
- Inflammatory diseases
- Dental complaints (also as a preventive measure)

Tip
Enzymes are available as tablets, creams, or enemas. For minor, external injuries, an enzyme cream will be sufficient. However, you can accelerate the healing process by taking enzyme tablets as well.

At this point, we would like to stress that under no circumstances should you treat an illness yourself. Enzyme preparations, as we will see later in more detail, can be immensely helpful for many complaints, but you should only use them if your doctor has given his or her approval. If you detect the first symptoms of an illness, don't put off the visit to your doctor, but seek his or her advice right away.

Similarly, don't be tempted to stop using a medication that you have been prescribed just because enzyme therapy has made you feel better. You would run the risk of a relapse and the illness becoming chronic.

We can't emphasize enough how important it is to seek and follow your doctor's advice if you suffer from a serious illness.

Medically Supervised Treatment

Nonprescription enzyme preparations shouldn't always be taken according to your own judgment, especially if they are to support conventional treatment such as a course of antibiotics. In these cases, it's important to consult your doctor.

Some enzyme preparations can only be obtained with a doctor's prescription—for example, those that are injected intravenously. Injected enzyme preparations are used as an aid for infusions and local anesthetics, for joint punctures, in gynecology, and in surgery.

Enzymes such as pancreatin and the digestive enzymes lipase and amylase must also only be taken under medical

Enzyme preparations can be obtained at pharmacies and health food stores.

If you are undergoing medical treatment, always consult your doctor if you are thinking of using a nonprescription enzyme preparation.

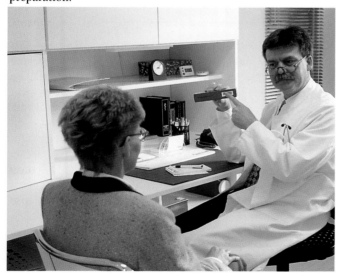

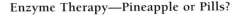

supervision. These enzymes are prescribed if the patient's pancreas isn't functioning properly and producing enough enzymes to break down food.

Cystic fibrosis is a very serious illness in which the secretion process of all glands is disturbed and the bronchial tubes are filled with glutinous mucus. It prevents nutrients from being absorbed in the intestine, and this is where enzymes can help to alleviate the symptoms. In addition, there are specific enzymes for chronic pulmonary diseases (chronic bronchitis and emphysema) that help to dissolve glutinous mucus.

In the case of an acute, life-threatening thrombosis, when a blood clot blocks an artery—for instance, in the leg—the enzymes streptokinase and urokinase can be injected intravenously.

Enzymes during pregnancy? As with other medications, these gentle remedies are best to be avoided during pregnancy. However, if a pregnant woman falls ill and could be treated with enzymes, then they might be preferable to conventional medications. As always, consult your ob-gyn first.

> ## When Enzymes Must Not Be Used
> - Chronic liver disorders
> - Chronic and advanced kidney disorders
> - Severe allergies, especially to proteins
> - Blood-clotting disorders
> - Hemophilia

Contraindications

People who suffer from blood-clotting disorders and hemophiliacs should never take proteolytic enzymes (bromelain, papain, trypsin, and chymotrypsin) and combined preparations. These enzymes cause the blood to become thinner, thus increasing the risk of severe bleeding in the case of an injury. Individuals who suffer from severe allergies should also be careful with enzyme preparations, especially if they are allergic to protein compounds. And patients suffering from acute pancreatitis must avoid enzyme treatments. Even if none of these contraindications applies to you, before you start taking any enzyme preparation always consult your own doctor.

One of Medicine's Most Powerful Weapons

Sports injuries, rheumatism, inflamed fallopian tubes, blood vessel disorders, toothache—enzymes help alleviate a range of complaints. What's more, they even play a role in diagnosing illness.

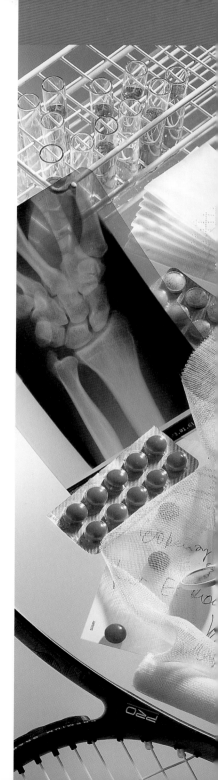

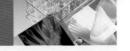

Painless and Precise: Diagnosis via Enzymes

At some time in your life, you have probably given a blood sample, which was analyzed in a laboratory. The result of the analysis, a long sequence of letters and numbers, doesn't usually mean much to the layperson. But we would like to shed some light on it, because these blood tests are closely related to our subject, the enzymes.

Laboratory Tests Reveal Enzyme Activity

Enzyme performance can easily be tested in the lab, because the enzymes are brought in contact with the substance that they are designed to break down. At intervals, measurements are taken as to how much of that substance has already been broken down.

As laboratory tests are improved and become increasingly sensitive, it has gotten to be possible to observe and measure enzyme activity in the blood very accurately. According to enzyme activity, the doctor can draw conclusions as to the nature of an illness and how it is likely to progress. Should the doctor observe that more enzymes than normal are active in the blood, this would indicate that there is an inflammation present somewhere in the body, because the immune system mobilizes more enzymes to remove diseased tissue. A lack of enzyme activity, on the other hand, would indicate a different kind of illness to the doctor—for instance, one in the digestive tract. The analysis of enzymes in the lab has thus become a reliable tool for recognizing the symptoms of an illness.

Alkaline Phosphatase (AP)

This enzyme occurs in the bones, the liver, the bile ducts, the lining of the small intestine, and, during pregnancy, in the placenta. If lab tests reveal an increased activity of alkaline phosphatase, this points to tumor metastases in the bones, hyperfunctioning of the parathyroid gland, or diseases of the liver or the bile ducts. Yet raised levels of AP are normal in growing children and in women in the third trimester of pregnancy.

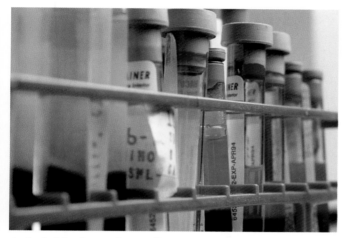

A single blood sample is sufficient to measure the levels of numerous enzymes and thus to examine various organs.

Alpha Amylase

This enzyme breaks down sugars and starches, and is produced in the pancreas and the parotid gland. If alpha amylase levels are raised, this could indicate a possible inflammation of the enzyme-producing glands. It is also possible that the exit ducts of the parotid gland or pancreas are defective.

Angiotensin I Converting Enzyme (ACE)

This stands for those enzymes that regulate blood pressure. They are considered an important indicator of a rare but usually treatable lung disorder called sarcoidosis (Boeck's disease).

Cholinesterase (CHE)

Cholinesterase gives away those who drink too much more than just occasionally. The CHE content of the blood is reduced dramatically if the cells of the liver are damaged or if there is cirrhosis of the liver. A CHE deficiency can also be genetic, or it can be caused by pesticides such as E605 and some insecticides.

Some enzymes break down diseased tissue and alleviate inflammation. An increased activity of these enzymes in the blood indicates that there is an illness somewhere in the body.

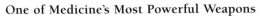

Creatin Kinase (CK)

This enzyme displays astonishing activity in the muscles of the heart and the skeleton. It is the first enzyme to show significantly raised levels in the blood as early as four hours after a heart attack. It is therefore a precise and life-saving indicator that a heart attack has taken place. Yet levels can also rise after strenuous exercise and other kinds of physical exertion as a result of muscular injuries and inflammation.

Gamma Glutamyl Transferase (Gamma GT)

Gamma GT can be found in the liver, the kidneys, the pancreas, the spleen, and the small intestine. Excessive amounts of this enzyme in the blood mean that the patient must avoid alcohol in order to put less strain on the liver. Possible causes for raised levels of gamma GT are a fatty liver due to excessive alcohol consumption, cirrhosis of the liver, and drug abuse, especially of sleeping pills, painkillers, or tranquilizers.

Always check whether or not your insurance covers a detailed enzyme analysis, because it is a fairly costly procedure and is usually done only if a specific illness is suspected.

Glutamate Dehydrogenase (GLDH)

This enzyme also indicates if there are problems with the liver. If GLDH levels in the blood are high, it is almost certain that liver cells are severely damaged. Occasionally, this is the result of poisoning, mainly through fungi and chemical cleaning agents.

With the help of glutamate-dehydrogenase (GLDH), doctors can measure the progress of viral hepatitis.

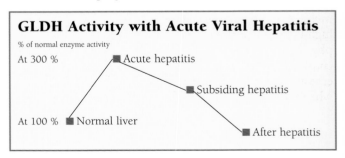

GLDH Activity with Acute Viral Hepatitis

% of normal enzyme activity

At 300 %   ◾ Acute hepatitis

◾ Subsiding hepatitis

At 100 % ◾ Normal liver

◾ After hepatitis

Glutamate Oxalacetate Transaminase (GOT)

GOT works in the muscles of the heart and the skeleton as well as in the liver. Like creatin kinase (see above), GOT is a reliable indicator of whether or not a patient has suffered a heart attack. A high concentration of the enzyme often also points to damage of or injuries to the skeleton.

Glutamate Pyruvate Transaminase (GPT)

GPT is another enzyme that provides information about infectious diseases of the liver. It is less active in the muscles of the heart and the skeleton; however, raised levels in these places can also indicate cell damage.

Lactate Dehydrogenase (LDH)

This enzyme can be found almost anywhere in the body's tissue. It is highly active in the heart muscle, the liver, the muscles of the skeleton, the red blood cells, and the blood platelets. LDH can indicate a heart attack up to eight to 10 days after the heart attack has taken place. This is especially useful if a heart attack has gone unnoticed and adverse effects don't occur until a few days later.

Lipase

This digestive enzyme breaks down fat and is produced in the pancreas. Its main place of work is the small intestine. Raised levels of lipase in the blood indicate an inflammation of the pancreas or a disease of the kidneys.

Phosphohexose Isomerase (PHI)

As an enzyme contained in the tissue, PHI in raised levels mainly indicates diseases of the tissue of the liver, the heart muscles, or the skeleton muscles. Levels are particularly high for acute hepatitis, heart attacks, and muscular dystrophy. With some kinds of cancer, PHI levels are monitored constantly for a better overview of the course that the disease and the treatment are taking. This is especially the case when it comes to bronchial, breast, and prostate cancer.

If your blood is to be analyzed for enzyme activity, you are not permitted to eat before you have your blood taken and may only drink water. Food would alter the enzyme levels, making the results of the enzyme test inaccurate.

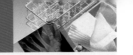

Sour Phosphatase (SP)

SP is mainly a male enzyme, as its highest levels by far can be found in the prostate. Smaller amounts can be found in the spleen, the bones, the red blood cells, and the blood platelets. Raised levels of SP can indicate prostate cancer or a possible bone tumor.

Just as the levels of individual enzymes can point to a particular illness, the sum of different enzyme concentrations or their relation to one another provides information as to which disease is more likely to be present. For this reason, GPT, GOT, Gamma GT, and GLDH levels are usually determined together.

Organs Examined by Enzyme Tests

Gallbladder and bile ducts	Alkaline phosphatase (AP)
Heart	Creatin kinase (CK) Glutamate oxalacetate transaminase (GOT) Lactate dehydrogenase (LDH) Phosphohexose isomerase (PHI)
Bones	Alkaline phosphatase (AP)
Liver	Cholinesterase (CHE) Gamma glutamyl transferase (Gamma GT) Glutamate dehydrogenase (GLDH) Glutamate pyruvate transaminase (GPT) Lactate dehydrogenase (LDH) Phosphohexose isomerase (PHI)
Pancreas	Alpha amylase Glutamate oxalacetate transaminase (GOT) Lipase
Prostate	Sour phosphatase (SP)
Muscles of the skeleton	Creatin kinase (CK) Glutamate pyruvate transaminase (GPT) Glutamate oxalacetate transaminase (GOT) Lactate dehydrogenase (LDH) Phosphohexose isomerase (PHI)

Invaluable in Treating Many Female Disorders

In terms of female disorders, enzyme therapy has already demonstrated three well-established areas of use: in the treatment of acute or chronic inflammation of the ovaries, the fallopian tubes, and the bladder, in postoperative aftercare, and in the treatment of benign changes in breast tissue (mastopathy). Enzyme therapy is also becoming of growing interest to women suffering from cancer. New results in this area can be expected within the next few years.

Changes in Breast Tissue (Mastopathy)

Practically all women will notice at some point in their lives that a gradual change has taken place in the shape and the size of their breasts. Frequently, women can feel small lumps in the breast tissue. In most cases, these changes are harmless. The lumps often turn out to be cysts, enlarged cavities of the ducts of the mammary gland, and real lumps generally end up being benign. Mastopathy can occur in one breast only or in both. Sometimes a fluid is secreted from the nipple. Painful breasts, however, are usually related to a woman's menstrual periods.

Even though mastopathy usually proves to be harmless and benign, it should not be taken lightly. A thorough examination by a doctor is advisable, especially because the symptoms of breast cancer are almost identical. The doctor will also feel the lump and, on the strength of that examination, decide whether or not further tests such as a mammogram or an ultrasound examination are necessary to verify the diagnosis. Only after the doctor has ruled out any possibly of the lump being malignant can enzyme therapy be started. But often the complaints are so minor that no treatment is necessary at all.

Tip
Seek the advice of your doctor or pharmacist regarding the different enzyme preparations. Multienzyme preparations containing pancreatin, bromelain, trypsin, papain, and chymotrypsin are best, because they have so many uses. Almost all of the disorders described here can be treated with these preparations.

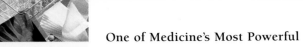

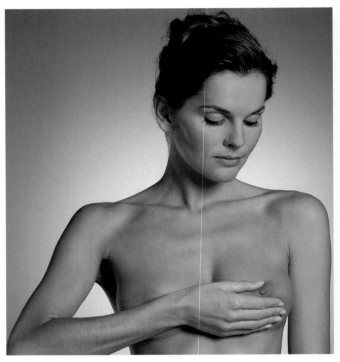

Examine your breasts once a month, and, if you discover any hardening of the breast tissue, any lumps, or other changes, see your doctor immediately.

An X-ray examination of the breasts, called a mammogram, is the most reliable method to date of discovering even the first initial stages of a small tumor. Not only does early detection increase the chances of curing the disease, but it also means that it is more likely that the breast will be saved, if surgery takes place early on.

Conventional Treatment

Again, we would like to emphasize that, without exception, you should never begin self-treatment without first consulting your doctor. For minor complaints, there are plant-based drops containing, for example, the active ingredients of black snakeroot, or cohosh. These substances have a similar effect in the body to that of progesterone. Should the symptoms be more serious, your doctor can prescribe creams containing hormones or, if there are no contraindications, hormone medications. In such cases, the doctor usually chooses medications with a high progesterone content, which the body normally produces itself naturally in the placenta and the ovaries.

54

The Effects of Enzymes

Recent experiments with enzyme therapy for mastopathy have shown remarkable results. In one study, after only six weeks of enzyme treatment, two-thirds of the patients were free of symptoms. The results were even better for those patients who had been given an additional vitamin-E supplement, with 85 percent of the patients showing no symptoms at all. Even an ultrasound examination could no longer detect any changes in breast tissue.

Professor Heinrich Wrba, a renowned Austrian enzyme researcher, observed that enzyme therapy combined with vitamin E causes mastopathy to disappear within three weeks and that no relapses occur later.

Yet women should not feel tempted to start enzyme therapy without consulting their doctors first, regardless of whether or not there is an increased risk of cancer. An exact diagnosis, at least by ultrasound and possibly by a mammogram as well, must precede any treatment. This is particularly important for women older than 30 years of age and where there is a history of cancer in the family.

Inflammation of the Fallopian Tubes

At swimming pools, on toilet seats, or during sexual contact, infectious germs have plenty of opportunity to enter the vagina and cause serious inflammation. Usually these germs are bacteria, which—as a worst-case scenario—can cause chronic illnesses that affect the entire pelvic area. Frequently a hospital stay is necessary for the sufferers.

Such complaints are very painful, and they greatly reduce the patient's ability to cope with stress and to work to her full potential. The symptoms include a suppurating discharge from the cervix and vagina, fever, and violent shivering. Laboratory results show an increase in the number of white blood cells, which means that the immune system is fighting the bacteria. The sedimentation test shows higher levels as well, indicating a serious illness. The best first-aid measure in such cases is strict bed rest.

Coffee, nicotine, and alcohol can exacerbate mastopathy pains. The pains can also be made worse by psychological problems and stress, as the breast tissue is very sensitive to mood changes and stressful situations.

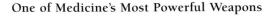

Conventional Treatment

In any case, the patient will require antibiotics and usually also some additional medication to reduce the swelling. These anti-inflammatory medications generally include corticosteroids, better known as steroids, in their active ingredients. Both types of medication should not be used over a long period of time because of their possible side effects.

Inflammation of the fallopian tubes requires urgent medical treatment. Should it become a chronic condition, the inflammation could have dangerous consequences, such as the formation of adhesions and scars, which could lead to infertility, and constant pain, which could permanently impair the patient's overall well-being. Apart from medication, it is advised to make use of physical measures like ice packs, radiation therapy (short-wave), and baths.

How Enzymes Can Help

Enzymes are particularly helpful in treating inflammations, where all their possible uses come to the fore. Enzymes can help in many different ways. In their function as "tugboats," they transport traditional medicines to their destination, thus accelerating and increasing their anti-inflammatory effect. In addition, enzymes remove the waste tissue that an inflammation invariably produces, causing healthy tissue to form faster, so that the inflammation often goes down much quicker. In this manner, enzyme therapy helps to prevent a dangerous, chronic inflammation of the fallopian tubes. It also reduces the swelling of the painful focus of the inflammation in the shortest possible time, lessening the pain simultaneously. As the blood values return to normal, it becomes apparent to the doctor that the enzyme therapy was successful and that serious, late aftereffects have been avoided. Therefore, if you are suffering from an inflammation of the fallopian tubes and are discussing treatment with your doctor, enzyme therapy should be considered as a possibility.

Lymphatic Edema

Lymphatic edema typically follows breast cancer treatment. The lymphatic vessels form a kind of drainage system in

With inflammation of the fallopian tubes, long-term enzyme therapy is definitely worthwhile. You should continue to take enzyme preparations for at least six months after an acute attack in order to prevent late aftereffects or a relapse.

the body through which lymph fluid transports the body's waste products away. In the lymph nodes, important immune reactions take place, such as trapping germs and rendering them harmless. If breast cancer also affects the lymphatic system, the cells of the tumor will cause it to cease functioning. Lymph will start to collect, thereby disabling an important function of the immune system. Lymphatic congestion damages the valves and the walls of the lymphatic system that regulate lymphatic flow. This causes inflammation, which in turn results in the swelling of tissue and exacerbates lymphatic congestion—a very dangerous cycle. Medical science distinguishes four stages of lymphatic edema:

- Latent (unobtrusive)
- Reversible
- Irreversible
- The stage called elephantiasis, in which the limbs become severely swollen

Conventional Treatment

The most important measure during the last stage is to raise the swollen limbs to an elevated position in order to encourage lymphatic drainage. The doctor will prescribe diuretic medicines and preparations for the veins. Pressure bandages and lymphatic massage are helpful too. The results of these measures, however, are usually not very satisfactory, and even surgery will only achieve limited success with advanced lymphatic edema.

How Enzymes Can Help

A study by the University Hospital in Prague shows that enzyme preparations improved the patients' condition significantly after only two weeks of treatment. The study was conducted with patients who had to have the entire breast and the lymph nodes removed surgically and, as a result, developed severe lymphatic edema. The effect of the enzymes here is similar to the way in which they work against inflammation. The Prague study recommends beginning enzyme therapy immediately after surgery, in order to prevent the lymphatic edema from becoming irre-

The effect of enzyme tablets in alleviating lymphatic edema can be reinforced by applying an enzyme cream.

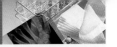

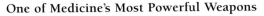

versible. A further benefit of enzyme therapy that is not mentioned in the study is that enzymes will also accelerate the healing process after surgery.

Endometriosis

This is a condition in which the lining of the uterus (the endometrium) grows outside the uterus instead of inside, but still within the genital area. Scattered parts can be found in the ovaries, the cervix, the vagina, the labia, and so forth. These scattered fragments of uterus lining form small blood-filled cysts that expand and grow continuously, because the blood cannot drain away. From the onset, endometriosis causes severe discomfort during menstruation and sexual intercourse.

It is estimated that about 8 to 10 percent of all women suffer from endometriosis. The greatest accompanying risk of the condition consists of adhesions and scars in the abdomen. These scars can cause lifelong problems, and there is a great risk of infertility if the endometrium grows and causes adhesions inside the fallopian tubes, as this would result in the ovum not being able to travel to the uterus.

Conventional Treatment

Endometriosis does not always require treatment. It depends on whether it causes pain or not. Treatment is advisable if a woman wishes to become pregnant. In serious cases, the doctor can use hormones (gestagens and antigonadotropins) to bring a halt to endometriosis. However, this hormonal treatment often comes with side effects, as it can cause complaints similar to those that occur during menopause. The side effects disappear once the medication has been stopped. The patient must not become pregnant during this treatment.

Women between 30 and 50 years of age sometimes suffer from a particular kind of endometriosis in which the lining of the uterus grows into the uterus muscles. This causes severe menstrual problems, and the uterus may even become slightly enlarged. In this case, the only solution is surgery.

Some female ailments have hormonal and psychosomatic causes. In these cases, enzyme therapy is unable to help. This is why irregular periods and PMS cannot be treated with enzymes, and neither can menopause. All enzymes can do is help a woman's overall well-being by improving the metabolism.

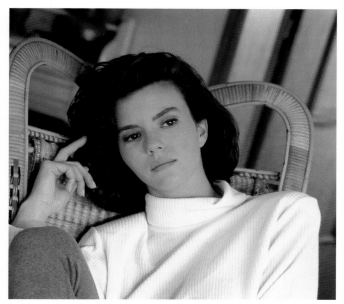

You don't need to fear abdominal surgery, as enzymes can reduce the severe pain and accelerate the healing process.

Studies have shown that, with endometriosis, the focus of the inflammation can be successfully eliminated if enzyme therapy supports conventional treatment.

How Enzymes Can Help

Especially with surgery, enzymes have proven beneficial as an accompanying therapy. Not only do they encourage the healing process, but they also prevent the formation of adhesions. Even in less severe cases, enzymes help to avert adhesions, because they actively take part in breaking down the scattered fragments of uterus lining. They also work against the formation of new adhesions after surgery, because they strengthen the body's immune system.

Risk of Miscarriage

According to medical science, a miscarriage occurs when a pregnant woman loses the embryo before it becomes viable outside the uterus (that is, before the end of the twenty-eighth week of pregnancy). If a woman has already suffered two or three consecutive miscarriages, this is called "habitual miscarriage."

Unfortunately, miscarriages like these are far more common than one would think. Roughly a third of all first pregnancies end in miscarriage. Despite the sorrow that accompanies such a loss, there is some consolation, as subsequent pregnancies usually progress perfectly normally. There are numerous reasons for miscarriage, and often they are psychological—for instance, the woman may subconsciously not be ready for a baby or her partner may reject the idea of pregnancy. Stress at work can also have damaging effects, especially for women who have to work very hard during the first few weeks of their pregnancy.

Hormonal imbalances (such as a lack of progesterone) are among the most common medical causes of miscarriage. As a result, the lining of the uterus does not form fully. Other causes include an incompetent cervix, genetic defects, damaged sperm, deformities or adhesions in the uterus, infections, and metabolic disorders such as diabetes or thyroid problems. The first signs of a miscarriage usually are pains similar to those during labor and varying degrees of bleeding.

Enzymes don't play an important role in childbirth yet, with two exceptions: They encourage healing after injuries to the perineum or the vagina during childbirth, and they strengthen the immune system prior to the birth. They may also be beneficial for strengthening the whole body in general.

Conventional Treatment

Depending on the cause of the problem, different therapies may be advisable. If the problem is caused by an underlying illness, naturally this is the primary condition that should be treated. Bed rest and relaxation are always important measures. Often the patient benefits from a dose of hormones such as progesterone or estrogen. If the embryo is lost, a curettage (a surgical scraping) is frequently unavoidable.

How Enzymes Can Help

It is not yet clear scientifically how enzyme therapy could help in this area of medicine. The ob-gyn in charge would have to draw on his or her experience with enzyme therapy and knowledge about how enzymes work in general. It is likely that enzymes could strengthen immunological processes in the body of a pregnant woman. However, the size and the position of the uterus have to be correct, oth-

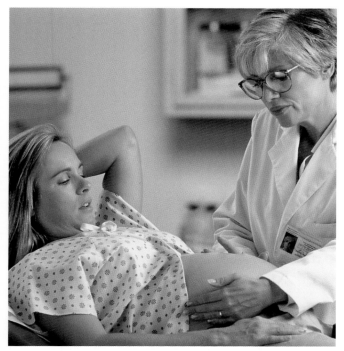

In problem pregnancies, enzymes can prevent the ovum from being rejected.

Tip
Enzyme therapy during pregnancy may be useful if the immune system needs to be boosted or there is a risk of miscarriage. However, even though existing research doesn't suggest that taking enzyme preparations during pregnancy causes deformities in the baby, these medications should be taken only with the doctor's consent.

erwise enzyme therapy—whether exclusive or supportive—will not be effective.

Bearing in mind the immunological effects that enzymes have, in women who display immune reactions to proteins, enzymes can be a major factor in stabilizing the immune system to such a degree that the body doesn't reject the ovum, which can then implant itself in the womb. Successful studies at the district hospital of Starnberg, Germany, support this theory. Major studies in this area have yet to be conducted, but it is certainly worth a try to save a baby by using enzyme therapy.

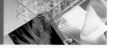

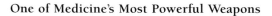

Vaginal Infections

Itchiness and a burning sensation in the vagina, a whitish or brownish-yellow discharge, pain, and sometimes even fever are the symptoms that should alert you to the possibility of a vaginal infection. The infection could be caused by bacteria, viruses, fungi, or trichomonads. Infections like these are usually transmitted during intercourse, but they can also be caught in unhygienic public bathrooms, saunas, and swimming pools.

In the case of vaginal infections, baths containing vinegar or herbal extracts can support enzyme treatment.

A smear allows the doctor to clearly identify the cause of a vaginal infection. At the same time, the doctor measures the acidity of the vaginal lining.

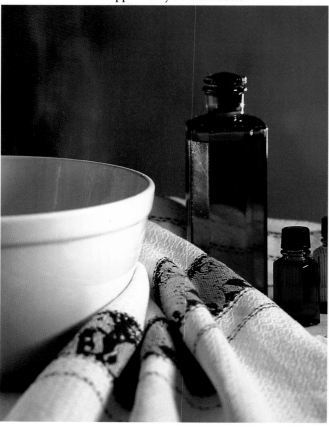

Fungal infections are drastically on the increase. This is partly due to exaggerated hygiene that damages the protective mechanisms of the skin, thus weakening the first important barrier of the body's immune system. In addition, fungal infections take a long time to be cured, so you can still infect your partner even when you think you are in the clear.

Chlamydiae are a particular kind of bacteria that is very easily transmitted during sexual intercourse. They cause a type of infection called chlamydia, which occurs more and more frequently these days. Chlamydia is very treacherous, because it often goes unnoticed. If the illness is not cured properly, however, it can lead to serious abdominal infections and, as a consequence, infertility. Trichomonads have a similar effect. These parasites cause trichomoniasis, an infection that occurs primarily in people who are promiscuous.

The symptoms of most vaginal infections are very similar, with those of a herpes infection being the exception. Three to seven days after the infection takes place (usually during intercourse), small, red blisters appear on the labia and around the vagina. These blisters are very itchy and cause severe pain. When they burst, they develop into small ulcers. The common assumption that, once you get herpes, you've got it for life, unfortunately is not far from the truth. Even though an initial herpes infection usually heals after a week, relapses occur frequently. Herpes cannot yet be cured completely. The virus simply hides in the body, ready to strike again at any time.

Tip
If one partner has caught an infection, the other partner should always undergo treatment as well. Otherwise the infection can travel back and forth like a Ping-Pong ball.

Conventional Treatment

Conventional medicine first determines what type of pathogen caused the infection. If it was caused by bacteria or trichomonads, antibiotics are usually the answer. This is also the case for chlamydia, the treatment of which can sometimes last up to four weeks. After a course of antibiotics, lactic acid suppositories should be prescribed to normalize pH levels in the vagina. Fungal infections are treated locally with creams, ointments, and vaginal suppositories. There are special medications for the herpes virus; some

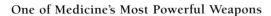

can be taken orally, whereas others are administered locally. Fungal infections require a great deal of patience, because they are difficult to cure completely. You can support the treatment yourself by taking warm hip baths:

- Fill a large hip bath with warm water (about 95 degrees Fahrenheit, or 35 degrees Celsius). For every quart, or liter, of water, add 2 tablespoons of vinegar. Bathe for approximately 15 minutes, and afterward take a cold shower. Then lie down and rest, covered warmly.
- Alternatively, prepare an infusion from chamomile or oak tree bark. Boil a quarter of the water required for the bath. Add 5 heaping tablespoons of your chosen herb per quart, or liter, of boiling water. Allow the infusion to cool, strain through a sieve, and add to the bathwater. Bathe for 15 minutes, take a cold shower, and rest, covered warmly.
- We recommend that you take a hip bath every night before going to bed.

How Enzymes Can Help

With infections that enter through the vagina, the greatest danger lies in the risk that germs may travel up into the pelvic area, causing serious infections with the possible consequences that were discussed earlier. Enzymes can counteract this because of their anti-inflammatory effect and their ability to accelerate the healing process. They encourage the immune system to fight the intruder fast. They also ensure the quick healing of wounds, thus preventing late aftereffects and chronic inflammation. Furthermore, enzymes provide general support for the immune system, as they stimulate its self-healing powers and support its fight against germs.

Cancer

The explanations below regarding enzyme therapy in the treatment of cancer are valid for all kinds of cancer, not just those specific to women such as breast cancer and tumors in the abdominal area.

The bad news first: Research to date has shown that enzyme therapy is of no use when trying to prevent cancer.

Tip
The correct dose is critical! With female disorders in particular, a high dosage of enzymes, taken consistently and without fail, is necessary for the first three to six months. So far, no side effects have been reported.

This is where vitamins, minerals, and a few other nutrients, such as vitamin E and C, beta-carotene, and selenium, can be helpful. However, in the treatment of cancer, there are some promising indications. The most significant studies on the subject were conducted by the renowned enzyme expert Max Wolf (1885 to 1976). His research into enzymes ultimately led to the development of the enzyme preparations available today.

A cancer cell, such as the one below, can be attacked by the specialists of the immune system. Enzymes support them in their work.

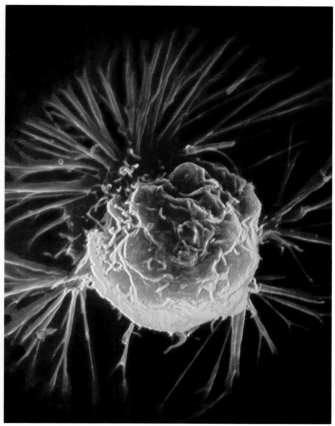

Max Wolf was the first to discover that enzymes are helpful in the battle against cancer. He is considered the founder of systemic enzyme therapy and has treated many famous patients in his New York practice, including the Kennedys, Pablo Picasso, Charlie Chaplin, Marilyn Monroe, and Marlene Dietrich.

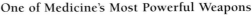

In the treatment of cancer, enzyme therapy is being used in an attempt to limit the growth potential of cancer cells or to destroy them altogether. Moreover, enzyme therapy has shown to be essential to freeing patients from the typical ramifications of the disease, such as weakness, loss of appetite, weight loss, and depression. These symptoms are directly linked to the weakness of the immune system.

Max Wolf therefore searched for the ideal medicine to combat cancer that would restrict the growth of the cancer cell while simultaneously strengthening the body's defenses and improving the patient's overall well-being. Research has shown that enzymes can at least strengthen the body's defenses without causing significant side effects. This means that enzyme therapy, like other biological therapies, is definitely of benefit in the aftercare of cancer patients.

Can Enzymes Kill Cancer Cells?

It seems that enzymes cannot fight the cancer itself. There is, unfortunately, still no substitute for traditional treatments such as surgery, chemotherapy, and radiation therapy. However, simultaneous enzyme therapy can support these harsh treatments by alleviating their side effects. Afterward, and particularly in the aftercare of surgery, enzymes can be given over a long period of time to strengthen the immune system and improve the patient's overall well-being.

Max Wolf did discover that certain enzymes have the ability to activate a cancer-destroying molecule formed by the immune system, the so-called tumor necrosis factor, or TNF. Enzymes such as bromelain, chymotrypsin, papain, asparaginase, and neuramidase could be of use for this purpose. There are other processes that have the ability to activate immune substances that can destroy cancer cells. Research as to how enzymes could take on a supporting function in these processes is being conducted presently. All of this, however, is still very much in the future.

Surgery Aftercare

Many women fear abdominal surgery, worrying about pain, complications, and possible late aftereffects. Of course, an

Clinical trials at the University Hospital in Homburg/Saar, Germany, have shown that treatment with multienzyme preparations greatly reduces the side effects of certain medicines used in chemotherapy. The positive effect of enzymes in this respect inspires hope for their use in the general treatment of cancer.

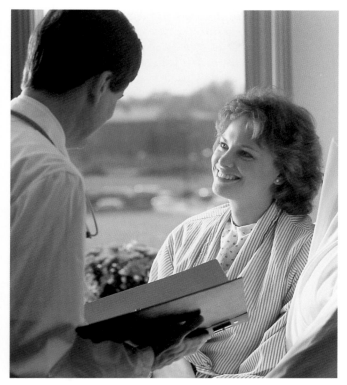

Enzyme preparations are being used more and more frequently to help patients regain their strength as soon as possible after surgery.

experienced surgeon will take the time to discuss all the risks with the patient prior to surgery, in order to allay any fears she may have, unfounded as they sometimes are.

Enzyme therapy after surgery, regardless of what type and on what organ, will ensure that wounds heal faster and inflammations die down more quickly. Therefore, the pain will be more bearable and will disappear sooner. Thanks to enzyme therapy, fewer problems occur during the recuperation period following surgery.

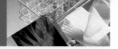

Enzymes Come to the Patient's Aid

The enzymes bromelain, trypsin, and the anti-inflammatory rutin (available as multienzyme preparations) reduce some of the risks that occur with surgery:

- The wounds caused by surgery are always accompanied by swelling and bruising. This slows down the healing process and thus increases the risk of infection and inflammation. Enzymes cause the swelling of tissue to go down, and they prevent bruising and transport waste tissue away. These are measures that improve the healing process and reduce pain.

- After every operation, there is a high risk of thrombosis, the formation of a blood clot that could block off a vital blood vessel completely. Surgery itself disturbs the blood circulation in the smallest blood vessels, and the risk is increased by the patients having to rest in bed. Enzymes, however, can improve the blood flow in the veins, so that even the smallest veins can receive a better blood supply again. Diseased tissue that has been freshly operated on requires a large amount of nutrients and oxygen to recover. If blood circulation is impaired, adequate supplies may be hampered.

Enzymes cause the blood to run thinner, so that it can transport nutrients essential to the healing process to even the finest capillary vessels, and it is better able to wash out waste products. If the power of the enzymes diminishes, the blood becomes thicker. This can result in deposits in the blood vessels, a weakening of the heart and circulation, or a disturbance of the blood supply. These are precisely the complications that may occur after major surgery. Therefore, surgery aftercare is one of the classic areas in which enzyme therapy is used. Numerous studies have proven that enzyme treatment encourages the healing process, thereby reducing pain.

Insurance companies benefit from enzyme therapy as well, because a faster recovery time means less time spent in the hospital, thus reducing cost.

Reliable Help for Many Other Complaints

Due to the wide range of applications that enzymes have for the body, female disorders are not the only area where they can be used successfully. Many other conditions that also affect men and children can be treated with the right enzyme preparation. In addition, enzymes can help prevent certain ailments and pain. It may therefore be advisable to take enzymes as a prophylactic measure.

When Enzymes Become Tired

The outbreak of some diseases, especially those that take a chronic course, can be traced back to a long-term enzyme deficiency in the body. This means the body cannot benefit from the protective and restoring effects that enzymes have. Enzyme activity usually slows down with age, making the body more susceptible to all sorts of vein complaints, such as phlebitis, thrombosis of the veins, and arteriosclerosis. A lack of enzymes can also be responsible for many age-related heart conditions, such as a weakened heart.

The less enzyme-friendly a life that someone has led, the earlier that conditions like vein complaints will appear. A lack of exercise slows down the metabolism and, with it, enzyme activity. A poor diet, low in raw fruit and vegetables, which contain a large amount of coenzymes, is another "sin against health."

Reduced enzyme activity also has a negative effect on the body's defenses, as they won't have the strength to fend off attackers such as viruses, bacteria, and fungi. A healthy immune system with plenty of active enzymes reacts strongly against intruders with, for instance, a fever. If these defense mechanisms are absent, it means that the immune system is weakened. All it would take would be an infection like the flu to cause persisting weakness, constant exhaustion, and a permanently reduced ability to

Among the most common complaints are minor injuries, suffered at home or when exercising. In these instances, the quick repair service that enzymes provide is invaluable. Enzymes aid healing, regardless of whether they are taken as a preventive measure or after the accident occurs. If you practice a dangerous sport, it may be in your best interest to always take enzyme preparations.

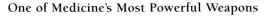

perform. You can recognize a weakened immune system, for example, by a persistent cold that is accompanied by poor immune reactions.

Suffering from Cancer—Yet Never Had the Flu?

A person who has rarely been sick with an infection and seldom run a fever is more likely to fall ill with cancer in old age. This is a discovery that the great enzyme expert Max Wolf made long ago, and it has recently been proven. A healthy immune system with active enzymes will cause the body to display very definite symptoms every time an infection takes hold. Antibodies and enzymes easily destroy individual cancer cells that are scattered throughout the body. However, if the immune system can't even fend off full-blown influenza, cancer cells will easily gain the upper hand against the weakened enzymes.

Preventive Care

When you first notice a weakness in your body's defenses, it is not too early to increase your enzyme intake and boost your immune system. Because there are almost no side effects to even long-term enzyme therapy and no adverse reactions with other medications, you can use enzymes yourself to prevent or treat the conditions described later in this chapter. If you suffer from a number of complaints, a multienzyme preparation might just do the trick for treating several symptoms at the same time.

Advice for Athletic Women

Exercise isn't all that important, some people say. These people usually prefer a more leisurely pace and are more interested in good food and alcohol. Smokers often fall into this category. There are some prominent exponents of this no-exercise way of life. Take, for example, the former British prime minister Sir Winston Churchill, who lived to a ripe old age of 91, despite his dislike of exercise.

Yet the exercising majority has the full backing of science and medicine. It is irrefutable that a certain amount of regular exercise keeps the heart, circulation, muscles, and joints healthy and young longer. Exercise also reduces

One ailment often attracts another. Chronic vein complaints, for instance, speed the development of arthrosis, and vice versa, because the pain that accompanies both conditions indicates that the patient does not get enough exercise. Enzymes can break into this vicious cycle. As they reduce swelling and inflammation and improve blood flow, they are able to alleviate both complaints at the same time.

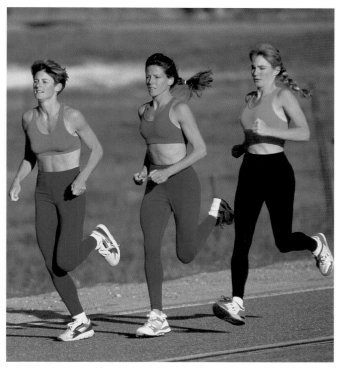

A study has shown that athletes who had pulled their ankle-joint tendons and were given enzyme treatment recovered on an average twice as quickly as those who did not receive enzymes.

Suffered a fall when jogging? Sprained your ankle? Minor sports injuries are no longer a problem with enzymes.

stress and can help prevent depressive moods to a certain extent. In addition, exercise encourages enzyme activity in the body, as it stimulates the metabolism and, with it, enzyme activity.

Risk of Injury

Unfortunately, exercise-related injuries are commonplace, occurring almost as often as accidents in the home. Professional athletes are not the only ones who suffer from such injuries—in fact, people who exercise in their spare time are the most at risk. Often they are eager to try trendy, new sports, but fail to prepare for them adequately or to train properly. They frequently don't warm up their muscles

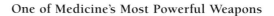

One of Medicine's Most Powerful Weapons

enough, and many also overestimate their level of fitness. In addition, amateurs don't always invest in the right equipment, which, however, is essential for safety.

High-Risk Sports

Some sports carry with them a particularly high risk of injury. Soccer, for instance, puts a lot of strain on knee joints, ankles, ligaments, and tendons. Skiing is notorious for broken bones and for pain from strained tendons and ligaments. With gymnastics and aerobics, you can easily sprain, bruise, and pull your muscles and ligaments. Trendy sports like bungee jumping and roller skating are especially high risk. If you prefer a pain-free way to fitness, try one of the more sedate sports. Swimming, cycling, jog-

External use of enzymes has proven to be extremely effective. Studies have shown that enzyme creams can speed up the healing of wounds by as much as 40 percent!

With minor external injuries, applying an enzyme-containing cream is very helpful.

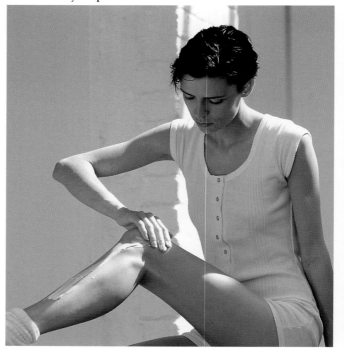

72

ging, and walking are the more risk-free ways of getting into shape.

When the Damage Is Done

There is a long list of common sports injuries, including sore muscles, muscle cramps, bruises, contusions, pulled muscles and tendons, sprains, and inflammations. Most of these injuries are very painful, some leaving a constant reminder of one's carelessness.

If you take enzymes immediately after sustaining an injury, you can avoid a lot of pain and shorten the healing process dramatically. The effect of the treatment will be the same as with the conditions discussed earlier: Enzymes will reduce the inflammation and the swelling, strengthen the immune system, and improve blood circulation. Also, edema and bruises will disappear more quickly, and pulled muscles and sprains will be less troublesome.

With grazes and lacerations, you can achieve an even better effect if you apply an enzyme cream in addition to taking enzymes internally. Yet enzyme therapy is no substitute for traditional first-aid measures at the scene of the accident such as cooling, compression, or, if necessary, putting the injured limb in an elevated position. Enzyme therapy can also possibly be used as a substitute for stronger medicines against pain, inflammation, and swelling, and thus spare you any unpleasant side effects.

Before an Accident Occurs

Enzymes are already being used to prevent sports injuries and their consequences. It has become quite common to give top athletes in basketball and football enzymes as a preventive measure. Enzymes optimize the function of the heart and circulation, make the immune system the strongest it has ever been, and help to prevent inflammation. And they are not considered illegal drugs! American boxing organizations instruct their boxers to take enzyme preparations in time for a fight, in order to prevent the consequences that boxing injuries normally incur. A study involving 100 hockey players has shown that swelling and pain are reduced much quicker if enzymes are taken pro-

Tip
Take enzyme preparations before you start your bodybuilding exercises, as this will prevent your muscles from becoming too sore.

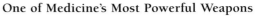
How to Reduce the Risk of Sports Injuries

Sport	Risk	Prevention
Cycling	Grazes, infection	Wear a helmet, be sure your tetanus immunization is up to date
Golf	Damage to the spine and shoulders	Learn and practice the correct technique
Gymnastics	Sprains, bruises, dislocation	Warm up muscles well, wear bandages to protect joints
Hiking	Carelessness is the greatest danger on your hikes	Buy quality equipment, consider using a guide
Horseback riding	Falls, back injuries	Exercises for the spine
Jogging	Exaggerated practice can result in heart and circulatory problems	Start slowly, wear loose clothing and supportive shoes
Skiing	Falls, broken bones, damage to tendons and ligaments	Special exercises designed for skiers; don't drink and ski
Soccer	Injuries to the knees, ligaments, tendons, and ankles	Exercises to warm up muscles
Squash	Sprains, pulled muscles and tendons, eye injuries	Use brightly colored balls, warm up properly
Swimming	Conjunctivitis, cramps in the calves	Wear goggles, take a magnesium supplement
Tennis	Same as squash; tennis elbow as well	Learn and practice the correct technique, wear the right type of shoes

Tip

Don't try to save money in the wrong area—make sure you have the right equipment for your sport! Hiking boots instead of sandals can prevent many an accident in the hills and mountains, the right tennis racket will be easier on your arm, and a safe bike will protect your bones and joints.

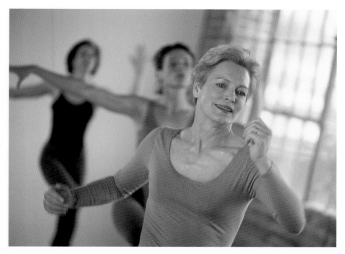

Warm up before you exercise. This will activate the body's enzymes and make muscles and joints more flexible.

Many people are treated for sports injuries, in the hospital or as out-patients.

phylactically: The swelling and pain disappeared within seven days, which is much faster than they would have without the enzymes.

Keep Exercising—Even If You're Older!
With age, injuries don't heal quite as quickly, and there is an increased risk of sustaining injuries through exercise because of age-related wear and tear in the body. Some older people can no longer quite master their sport technically, which means an increased risk of injuries and accidents. But this shouldn't be taken as a reason to give up sports when you are older—exercise is good for you, no matter what your age is! With increasing age, the flexibility and suppleness of muscles, bones, tendons, and ligaments are especially important. If you don't keep exercising, you will get stiff! And, by taking enzyme preparations, you can effectively prevent any major damage from occurring.

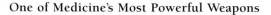

Preventing Varicose Veins

If you want to believe the media, then there are a whole array of miracle cures in the form of pills, creams, and lotions that make varicose veins disappear. The truth, however, is that surgery (sometimes very minor) is the only way to remove them. Therefore, you should try to prevent varicose veins from developing in the first place, and enzymes can assist you in this.

Initially, varicose veins are only a cosmetic problem. They appear as thick, winding blue veins, making you think twice about wearing panty hose or a short skirt. Later on, varicose veins can cause problems and lead to more serious vein disorders.

Veins—Extremely Hard Workers

As a rule, vein complaints are caused by a disturbance of the blood flow in the affected blood vessels. The function of the veins is to transport used blood, which is full of metabolic waste products, back to the heart. The walls of the veins are thinner, more elastic, and less muscular than those of the arteries, which transport fresh, oxygen-rich blood to every cell in the body.

The work of the veins, however, is much harder. They have to pump the blood against gravity up to the heart. So that the blood does not suddenly flow in the wrong direction, the veins are equipped with valves that prevent the blood from flowing back. Capillaries run between the veins and the arteries. They absorb used blood from the cells through their walls or supply fresh blood to the cells. The vein system has a very complicated and complex structure. The main vein transports blood to the heart. En route are numerous blood vessels of varying sizes that prevent a buildup of blood. There are three types of vein in the leg: those found directly below the skin, those found in the muscles, and those that connect the two others.

Different Vein Disorders
Varicose Veins

A vein in which a buildup of blood develops will no longer run in a straight line, but in a zigzag pattern. Varicose veins

> Your family doctor may not be the right person to consult regarding varicose veins. There are doctors who specialize in ailments concerning the veins called phlebologists, and they have the knowledge and the equipment necessary for gentle forms of diagnosis and therapy. Ask your doctor to refer you to such a specialist in your area.

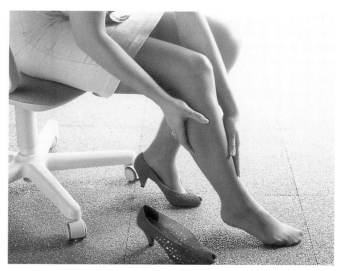

Do your best to keep your legs beautiful and smooth. Enzyme preparations can prevent varicose veins.

develop when one of the valves in the vein is no longer working properly. This will cause blood to build up in the vein, which in turn will cause the walls of the vein to stretch.

There are many kinds of varicose vein, some more dangerous than others. The so-called rose vein runs from the groin along the inside of the leg down to the ankle. It is located directly under the skin and is particularly at risk. This vein accounts for two-thirds of all visible varicose veins. If this important major vein is affected, medical treatment is necessary—otherwise, more vein problems will develop.

Skin Changes
Yellow or blue spots on the skin are a first sign of poor circulation. The skin also takes on a translucent quality, like parchment. Lying down in bed, you may suddenly have an unbearable itch on your leg, because the hormone histamine is activated by the poor blood circulation in the skin.

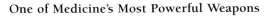

Phlebitis

Phlebitis always causes severe pain. The affected vein turns red, starts to swell, and becomes hot. In the case of phlebitis, there is a risk of developing thrombosis or even a pulmonary embolism. It is imperative that you seek medical treatment!

Thrombosis

This is the blocking of a vein by a blood clot. Thrombosis is dangerous, because it may go unnoticed for a long time, while the blood clot continues to grow until it blocks the vein completely. In the worst-case scenario, the blood clot becomes detached from the wall of the vein and travels along the bloodstream. It could end up in a pulmonary artery and block it, causing a pulmonary embolism, which is a potentially life-threatening condition. However, thrombosis doesn't always go unnoticed. It usually causes pain from the calf up to the groin, the leg begins to swell, and the symptoms are often accompanied by fever.

Leg Ulcers

Ulcers on the calf are one of the most persistent and difficult-to-heal vein ailments there are. They can be caused by untreated thrombosis. If a blood clot attaches itself permanently to the wall of a vein, a constant buildup of blood results, making it more difficult for waste products to be transported away. As a result, brown patches and inflammation develop, cells die, and an ulcer forms.

What Causes Vein Disorders?

Women struggle with vein ailments more than men do. Contrary to widespread belief, this is not the result of women becoming pregnant. In fact, only 30 percent of women develop varicose veins after the first child, and 55 percent develop varicose veins only after several children. Compared to men, however, women frequently have a genetic predisposition to weak connective tissue or vein disorders. Veins, in particular, depend on a strong connective tissue to support them adequately, because they have very thin walls and practically no muscles of their own.

Tips
You can prevent varicose veins to a certain extent by walking a lot, putting your feet up whenever possible, and alternating hot-and-cold water rapidly when you shower. All this improves circulation in the legs and means that more enzymes are made available to help keep vein problems from developing.

In addition to genetic predisposition, the major causes of vein disorders are a lack of exercise, a one-sided diet, being overweight, smoking, and the consumption of alcohol. A high-calorie, high-fat diet and the resulting excess weight put a lot of strain on the legs and the veins. A poor diet also means a sluggish digestive tract and poor digestion. The result is an inefficient metabolism that can no longer remove cell waste effectively.

Prevention: Better Than Any Medication

Medication for your veins, whether for external or internal use, will not achieve very much on its own. You will have to contribute your share as well. Eating healthy meals consisting of raw vegetables and fruit, salads, and plenty of whole-grain products will improve bowel function. Take regular walks, go on hikes, or participate in other sports that depend on your legs. Lymphatic drainage and oxygen therapy can also be beneficial.

How Enzymes Can Help

To what extent can enzymes help alleviate vein disorders? They develop their full potential if they are activated at the first sign of a vein problem. Once the problem becomes established, even enzymes are only able to support other treatments that your doctor will prescribe. Enzymes really come into their own if used as a preventive measure or in the very early stages of the vein disorder.

Deposits Don't Stand a Chance

At the first attempt of blood fat and calcium combining to form a blood clot, our enzymes appear on the scene. If they reach the problem area soon enough, they can prevent the buildup of deposits by transporting the blood clot away. If a blood clot has attached itself to the wall of a vein but is still quite small, enzymes are able to dissolve it and remove the debris.

Thinner Blood Flows Better

In order for blood clots to form in the first place, a substance called fibrin is necessary. Fibrin occurs in the blood-

Tips
The majority of people today work in offices, sitting behind a desk. If you are one of these people, try to compensate for being stationary for such a large portion of your day by climbing the stairs instead of taking the elevator or by parking your car a block or two away from your office and walking the rest of the way. Daily exercise in fresh air will also benefit your veins.

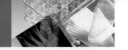

stream, and, without it, it would be impossible for blood platelets to stick together and form blood clots. This is where enzymes are useful: They remove excess fibrin, while at the same time aid in the normal clotting of blood. All three factors combined—clotting, removal of fibrin, and dissolving of blood clots—improve blood flow.

Leg Ulcers and Enzymes

The three most important qualities of enzymes also support the effective treatment of leg ulcers. Enzymes remove cell and metabolic waste from the wound, ensure that the supply of nutrients to the diseased tissue is improved, and improve blood circulation.

If It's Good for Circulation, It's Good for the Heart

Many people suffer heart attacks, and a significant proportion die from them. In the United States, one and a half million people have a heart attack each year.

No other organ in the body works as hard as the heart muscle. The motor that keeps us going beats a hundred thousand times a day, without respite, and several billion times throughout our lives. But the way we live today makes the work of our most important organ much more difficult. Blood vessels suffer as they become less elastic and clogged with deposits. As a result, the heart has to work harder and harder in order to fulfill its original task. Irregularities in the functioning of the heart are always followed by other complaints, as the oxygen supply of the whole body is jeopardized.

There are warning signs that the heart may be under too much strain: breathlessness when walking briskly or climbing stairs; a bluish tint to lips, toes, and fingers; arrhythmia; and pains in the region of the heart, which includes the arms, back, and chest.

Everything that enzymes can do for blood circulation will also be beneficial for the heart. They will improve blood flow, prevent deposits and the narrowing of veins, and generally increase the oxygen supply to the blood. For all these reasons, enzymes are an important medication in the prevention of heart attacks.

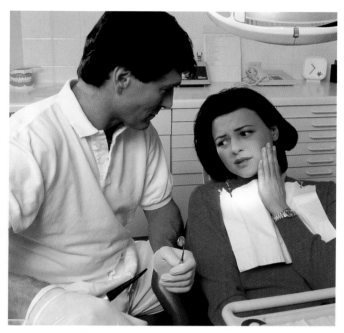

You don't need to be concerned about getting a swollen cheek after a tooth has been extracted, because enzyme tablets will reduce the risk of swelling.

No More Fear of the Dentist

Where dental treatment is concerned—the pulling of teeth, oral surgery, implants, root canal, and surgery to install dentures—enzymes help in a way that is similar to enzyme treatment with other surgery. Yet there may be a greater need for them here, as all oral surgery causes more severe swelling and pain than surgery elsewhere. This is due to the fact that the blood supply to the lining of the mouth is much greater than in other parts of the body, and, where there is more blood, more severe swelling and pain develop. In addition, a dentist usually only gives a local anesthetic, which doesn't last as long as a general anesthetic, and so you will feel the dreaded pain after the surgery all the sooner.

Tip
How you can help yourself following dental treatment: Apply an ice pack to the swelling, and take a high dosage of an enzyme preparation that contains both plant- and animal-based enzymes. The numerous effects that enzymes have on a wound will also help to alleviate pain and possibly save you from having to use a stronger medication.

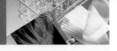

What Exactly Is Swelling?

Every injury to the body initially causes swelling. This is a sensible protective measure by the body. A swelling does the same as we do to stem blood flow—namely, compresses blood vessels so that the wound will not bleed for too long. Unfortunately, in most cases, the swelling remains for longer than is necessary to stem the blood flow and thus impedes the healing process.

Simply put, a swelling consists of protein molecules that have transferred from the blood into the tissue. Once their work is done, however, they need to be removed from the tissue, otherwise the swelling won't go down. A swelling also causes pain, as it continuously applies pressure to sensitive nerve endings.

Tip

If your fear of the dentist is to the extent of a phobia, you might want to consider a hospital for major dental surgery. There, you will receive medical care both before and after the surgery.

What Else Impedes the Healing Process?

Dental surgery is accompanied by the same risks as all other surgery. The main risks are bruising and poor blood supply. There is also a danger that blood clots and inflammation may develop. All of the above hinder the healing process significantly, but poor circulation and swelling are the main culprits. In addition to being painful, they are also annoying because they mean that you will have a swollen cheek for a few days.

Which Enzymes Are Recommended?

The most common, prescription-free multienzyme preparations contain both plant-based enzymes (bromelain and papain) and animal-based enzymes (trypsin and chymotrypsin). This combination of enzymes is the most useful after dental surgery, utilizing the same active ingredients that are used for all conditions that entail inflammation, swelling, and pain.

A Faster Route to Recovery

Once enzymes are taken, the wound will heal in a matter of days. Without enzymes, a wound will heal very slowly, as the supply of nutrients and oxygen is disturbed because of a poor blood supply. In addition, the buildup of blood prevents waste products from being removed. There is also a danger that pathogens may enter a slowly healing wound. Yet another challenge for our enzymes! So, if you plan to have dental surgery, it is advisable to take enzyme preparations two or three days before the operation in order to prevent severe swelling, pain, and inflammation.

Rheumatism

Rheumatism almost falls under the category of female disorders these days, as it affects twice as many women as men. Rheumatism rarely affects children, but when it does, the symptoms are much more severe. There are more than 100 different conditions that can be classified as a type of rheumatic disease. Yet the term "rheumatism" can sometimes be misleading, because many of the conditions that we are quick to call rheumatism are actually not of rheumatic origin.

For instance, it is a common error to regard gout as a rheumatic disease. Although it is true that gout also affects the joints and especially those of the big toes, it is originally a disturbance of the purine metabolism. Gout requires an exact diagnosis by your doctor and subsequent careful treatment. It is correctly referred to as a disease of luxury, as its main cause lies in consuming too much rich food and alcohol. As a result, uric acid, which can no longer be flushed out by way of the kidneys, is deposited in the form of tiny crystals in joints, cartilage, skin, and the renal pelvis. However, taking enzymes will have little effect on gout—abstaining from rich, high-calorie food and from alcohol completely is the most effective form of treatment.

Minor Complaint or Rheumatism?

Everybody is sometimes plagued by pains in the joints and the muscles. There may be a pain in the shoulder, twinges in the hand or knee joints, or suddenly a touch of lumbago in the back. Occasional complaints like these are perfectly normal, especially if your job is very demanding, if you are continuously lifting small children, or if you were careless when exercising. If you think about what you have been doing, usually the source of these complaints is not hard to identify. Joint and muscle pains often also occur as a symptom of a cold or other infection.

Tip
Enzyme therapy for rheumatism requires a little patience. However, if your condition has not improved after six weeks, ask your doctor whether you should increase your enzyme dose or start taking enzymes by injection, which will have a much more powerful effect.

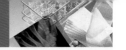

In these instances, it helps to go easy on the affected joint and apply creams that improve blood circulation. It is also advised to support this treatment with enzyme therapy.

A Short Checklist for Your Joints

- Do you frequently suffer from pain without an apparent cause?
- Does the pain affect the same joint all the time?
- Do you feel stiff in the morning and find it difficult to move your limbs properly?
- Do you notice swelling of individual joints? Do they feel hot, and are they red?
- Apart from the pain in your joints, do you sometimes have a fever or a lack of appetite?
- Do you avoid certain movements or types of exercise, because you fear they might cause you pain?

Tip
Sometimes the nerves are responsible. If you feel constant tension in your arms, legs, shoulders, or neck, your nerves may be overwrought. Relaxation, warmth, simple loosening-up exercises, and gentle massage may all be helpful.

If one or more of the above apply to you, consult your doctor right away to establish whether or not you are suffering from a rheumatic disorder. If you take recurring pains in your muscles and joints lightly, you run the risk of one day being limited in your mobility or constantly having to live with a certain degree of pain. X rays and a blood test can determine the precise source of your pain.

If the pain is severe, it is definitely recommended to take traditional medications prescribed by your doctor, in order to avoid entering a vicious cycle of pain and ever-decreasing mobility. Pain causes us to go easy on the affected joint, but to tense it at the same time—and this will only cause further problems.

The Most Common Rheumatic Disorders
The most painful and common form of rheumatism is chronic polyarthritis, which can occur at any age. Just as common is degenerative rheumatism of the joints, in which the joints are worn and cause pain. Another type of rheumatism, the so-called rheumatism of the soft parts, mainly affects muscles, nerves, and tendons.

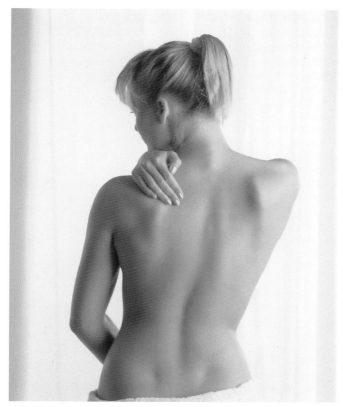

Tip
Acute polyarthritis has become rarer. It develops from a bacterial infection with streptococci, which today can easily be treated with antibiotics.

Check your joints regularly, and consult your doctor if you experience recurring pain in certain joints.

The Most Common Causes of Rheumatism

- One-sided movements executed regularly over a long period of time
- Tension due to excessive strain on the nerves
- Thickening of bones
- Weight gain, causing increased strain on the bones
- Wear (rarer)
- Genetic predisposition
- Immune deficiency

Chronic Polyarthritis

This illness is also referred to as "rheumatoid arthritis" or, if it occurs in children, as "juvenile arthritis." Unfortunately, it starts with very unspecific symptoms before the pain in the joints even sets in. Patients suffer from a recurring mild fever, along with a lack of appetite and a resulting weight loss. Soon afterward, the inflammation starts in the finger joints. This is followed by attacks in the joints of the hands, feet, knees, and hips. The chronic inflammation in the individual joints not only causes excruciating pain, but it also gradually destroys the cartilage, resulting in the joints' becoming stiff and deformed.

When the Body Becomes Self-destructive

Chronic polyarthritis is caused by a malfunction of the body's immune system. Instead of attacking invading pathogens, the immune system attacks the body. Chronic polyarthritis is the most common autoimmune disease. The same malfunction of the immune system also causes other, equally devastating diseases such as multiple sclerosis and the bowel disorders Crohn's disease and ulcerative colitis.

What is happening here? Our immune specialists are suddenly attacking the body's own healthy cells for some unknown reason. The antibodies attach themselves to an enemy and form immune complexes. Once these float in the blood, they are destroyed by the macrophages. If they have attached themselves to body tissue, they can only be annihilated by the complementary system, with the result that healthy tissue is eliminated as well.

We can picture only too easily what happens in an organ or other part of the body where the body's own immune system is running riot. The macrophages constantly form new immune complexes and lodge them in the tissue, and the complementary system continues to destroy them and, with them, more and more healthy tissue. The organ that is thus attacked reacts with severe inflammation, swelling, and fever—it's an endless battle fought by the immune system.

The immune complexes in which the antibodies enter with the body's own protein molecules are referred to as "disease-causing immune complexes." They can be detected in the blood and back up the diagnosis of chronic polyarthritis.

A Real Challenge for Medical Science

Medical science has so far failed to discover how to effectively end this battle in the body and stop the destruction of an entire organ. The only option to date is to immobilize the immune system completely by using so-called immune suppressives. These medications, of course, have serious side effects. If the immune system is no longer working, every single germ or each common cold potentially endangers the life of the patient.

Enzyme therapy, however, has given a justified rise to fresh hope in treating chronic polyarthritis, because enzymes can break down the immune complexes that cause the problem. Initial patient studies showed that pain and inflammation were considerably reduced. Some patients were also able to decrease the dose of their regular medication significantly and thus suffered less of the often serious side effects that traditional rheumatism medicines can cause. It is true that enzyme therapy is successful in only 50 percent of polyarthritis cases, but traditional treatments do not have a higher success rate.

Arthrosis

This degenerative condition is characterized by wear and tear of the joints and can affect anyone more than 40 years of age. It is not clear, however, why some people seem to be completely unaffected by the wear in their joints, whereas others suffer from severe pain and greatly restricted mobility.

Arthrosis mainly affects the hip and knee joints. At first, it attacks the layer of cartilage within the joint. In young people, this layer covers the entire joint, so that the joint can move smoothly in the way it was intended. With age, the layer of cartilage becomes brittle, because constant movement has gradually worn it down.

Now the painful part of the illness begins. Pieces of cartilage fall off and into the gaps between the joints. This causes friction and irritation with every movement, resulting in severe pain, swelling, and occasionally inflammation of the affected joint.

Bechterew's disease is a rare rheumatic disease characterized by chronic inflammation of the joints of the spine. It is not clear what brings about this condition; both genetic predisposition and an infection (viral or bacterial) are possible causes.

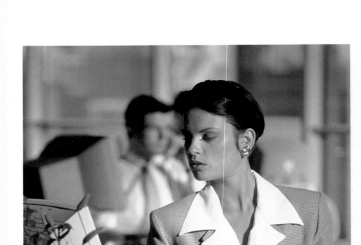

Cartilage in the joints—
for example, in the knee—
cannot be restored once it
has been destroyed. Even
enzymes are unable to
help in this respect. Yet
enzymes can alleviate the
excruciating pain.

Many people who suffer from tennis elbow subject their arms
to a certain type of repetitive movement, for example, by
working with a computer.

No Remedy for Wear

Once the cartilage has been damaged, medical science can't
do anything to reverse the process. Only in the later stages
of the disease will surgery be considered to replace the
affected joint with an artificial one. The treatment with traditional medications mainly aims at alleviating pain, preventing possible inflammation, reducing swelling, and
keeping the joint mobile as long as possible.

Rheumatism of the Soft Parts

As the name suggests, this disorder affects the soft parts of
the structure that enable us to move—that is, the muscles,

the tendons, the ligaments, the mucous membranes, and the nerves.

A typical example of this kind of disorder is what is known as "tennis elbow." However, the name of the condition is somewhat misleading, because, along with tennis players, it frequently affects people who may have never held a tennis racket in their lives, such as typists, housewives, or people working with some kind or machinery. Continuous, repetitive movements such as typing and ironing can bring about the disorder, causing severe pain in the elbow. It is there that the tendons of the forearm extensor end, and it is these tendons that are under excessive strain because of the constant, monotonous movements.

Another typical example of rheumatism of the soft parts is what is known as "acute shoulder," in which every attempt to move the arm is accompanied by unbearable pain in the shoulder joint. This can either be caused by an inflammation of the tendon or by calcification of the mucous bursa. "Secretary's disease," or tendinitis, also falls in this category.

With rheumatism of the soft parts, patients themselves are often responsible for their condition. If you subject certain parts of your body to long-term, excessive strain, be it through exercise or work, don't be surprised if symptoms of wear occur some months or even years down the line.

Self-help for Minor Rheumatic Complaints

The physical and plant-based therapies discussed below are well suited to effectively support conventional medical treatment and reduce rheumatic pain. You may even be able to decrease the dosage of the medicines your doctor has prescribed for pain, swelling, and inflammation. However, don't make any changes in your treatment without consulting your doctor first.

Protection or Exercise

If you suffer from either rheumatism of the soft parts or arthrosis, initially you must avoid any movement that puts strain on the affected part. The opposite is true for chronic polyarthritis. In this case, you can learn gentle exercises

Tip
If you suspect you may be suffering from a rheumatic disorder, you should consult your family doctor or a specialist in internal medicine without delay. Many hospitals also have rheumatism clinics where you can seek advice.

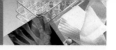

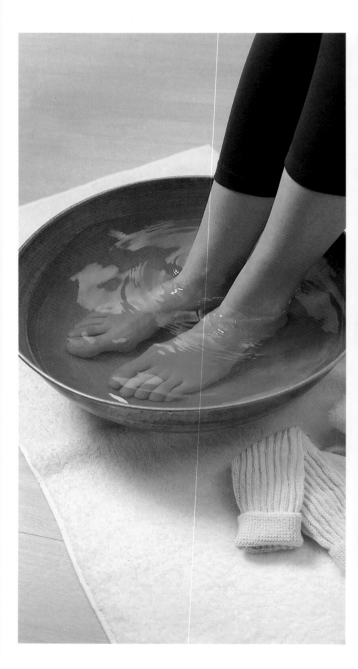

Tip
Support your rheumatism treatment with Kneipp's water therapies, such as footbaths or pouring water over parts of your body (see pages 111 and 112).

that will alleviate pain in the long term by making the joint more mobile. This will prevent the joint from stiffening, which would result in increased pain.

Hot and Cold Compresses
Hot compresses relieve pain and relax the muscles. Both hot and cold compresses have an anti-inflammatory effect to a certain extent, but cold compresses have the additional advantage of improving circulation and thus promote the healing process.

Baths with Plant Extracts
A relaxing bath enriched with the right plant extracts can relax muscles and reduce pain. Bath additives with juniper oil or with salicylates obtained from willow tree bark are particularly beneficial. You should be able to purchase these from your pharmacy or health food store. Seek advice from the salesperson, and follow the instructions on the package.

Herbal Teas
You can buy special herbal teas that foster the treatment of rheumatism. They are available from a number of manu-facturers and different outlets. Typically, they contain the following ingredients:
• Rampion, which improves the removal of waste prod-ucts from the metabolism
• Juniper, which is particularly helpful against arthrosis
• Willow tree bark, which has anti-inflammatory proper-ties
• Echinacea, which improves the body's overall self-healing ability

Enzymes Give Rheumatism Sufferers Hope
As rheumatism can thus far only be treated according to its symptoms, patients are faced with long-term therapy. Medications have to be taken over a long period of time, which lends particular significance to the questions of side effects, interaction with other medications, and general tol-erance, as well as cost.

Tip
Rheumatic disorders require a whole array of medical measures. Enzymes are well suited to complement these measures, because they don't interact with other medicines.

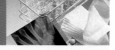

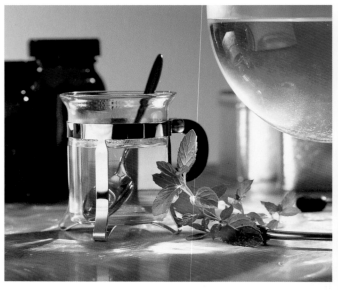

Add 3 teaspoons of the above herbs to 1 quart, or liter, of boiling water. Let the tea steep for 10 minutes.

Tip
Strictly speaking, there is no rheumatism diet. However, a sensible diet that improves metabolic function, assists in the removal of waste products, and strengthens the immune system can have a positive influence on the healing process. A high-quality diet in which foods are as close as possible to their natural state is best. A sensible diet is an enzyme-friendly diet that ensures that the little biological helpers are supplied sufficiently with coenzymes.

Several studies over the last few years have proven how effective the use of enzymes can be in the treatment of rheumatic disorders. One study looked at 43 men and 37 women between 18 and 80 years of age who were suffering from arthrosis in the knee joint. Half of them were given conventional rheumatism medicines, whereas the other half were given an enzyme preparation. After two weeks and again after four weeks, the group that had taken the enzyme preparations surprisingly had made very similar progress compared to the group that had taken the conventional remedies.

Which enzymes are helpful in treating rheumatism? Rheumatism of the soft parts and arthrosis are best treated with trypsin, bromelain, and papain, whereas chronic polyarthritis responds best to a combination of trypsin, bromelain, and rutin. When treating rheumatic disorders with enzymes, their most important properties will take effect.

Enzymes against Inflammation?

Inflammation is always a sure sign that there is something wrong with the tissue of the affected organ. It either means that a pathogen has entered or that there is a defect in the tissue itself, such as a wound or an autoimmune reaction. In all instances, the tissue uses defensive measures in order to restore its normal healthy state as quickly as possible. First, it releases the tissue hormone histamine, which will transport more blood to the focus of the illness and activate the antibodies of the immune system. In the case of an autoimmune disease, in which the immune system attacks the body, this is entirely the wrong course of action, encouraging an utterly senseless defense reaction.

The inflamed area then swells due to the increased blood supply and, on the outside, becomes red and hot to the touch. In the meantime, enzymes have reached their destination and gotten busy removing dead tissue, waste products, and so forth. A number of molecules participate in this process.

Therefore, it can be said that an inflammation is initially a sensible reaction by the immune system to pathological changes in the tissue. But often an inflammation persists for longer than necessary, causing the patient more pain.

Enzymes are capable of shortening this process gently by helping to improve the blood supply and providing the damaged tissue with fresh nutrients. They break down the protein molecules that are responsible for the swelling. Enzymes may not work quite as quickly as synthetic anti-inflammatory drugs, but they are just as effective and don't have any of the side effects that accompany the conventional remedies, such as high blood pressure, stomach ulcers, kidney disease, thrombosis, and depression. The longer these medicines are taken, the more these side effects occur.

Initially, an inflammation is a sensible reaction by the immune system. However, it must not last for too long—as is the case with chronic illnesses—as it would then impede the healing process.

Harmful Immune Complexes

According to the research that has been conducted thus far, enzymes are capable of something that none of the other medications used in the treatment of chronic polyarthritis can achieve. They are able to remove from the tissue those

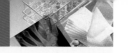

harmful immune complexes that cause the disease to progress further and further. Only when the immune complexes have been removed from the affected tissue will the excessive reaction of the immune system cease. Once they are removed, the immune complexes enter the bloodstream, where other members of the defense troops can dispose of them easily.

Enzymes—and Nothing Else?
In a few cases, enzymes are sufficient as the sole medication for long-term therapy. However, when the treatment begins and the patient is suffering from severe pain and is restricted in mobility, conventional rheumatism medications are an absolute necessity. But it's still a big step forward if enzyme preparations can help to reduce the dosage of these medications in the long term and thus significantly decrease their side effects. The greatest advantage of enzymes, apart from the effects they have, lies in the fact that, in contrast to other medications, they don't have any undesired, harmful effects on your health.

Gold Therapy—the Other Side of the Coin
If you are constantly suffering from severe arthritic pain, you are probably willing to try anything that might help. For this reason, every now and then, gold therapy comes up as a possible treatment for chronic polyarthritis. It is undeniable that it has produced good results in about 50 percent of the cases—but at what price! The organic gold compounds, in the form of tablets, damage the stomach and the bowels and, in many patients, have caused severe inflammation of the skin accompanied by pain and itching. Damage to internal organs cannot be ruled out either.

The Section for Him: Prostate Complaints
Men don't like to talk about prostate complaints, which is understandable. But if you notice that your husband or partner seems to have a loss of libido and is going to the toilet much more frequently than usual, he could have a prostate problem. Also, prostate complaints are often accompanied by varying degrees of pain.

Tip
When it comes to taking enzyme preparations for rheumatic disorders, the success of the treatment depends to a large extent on the right dosage. The amounts recommended in the printed matter that comes with the medication aren't always right for each individual case. Therefore, discuss the dosage with your doctor, or consult the manufacturer of the medication.

Warning Signs for Prostate Problems
- He complains that he needs to go to the toilet constantly.
- Urinating causes him pain.
- The urine stream is reduced to dripping.
- He needs to get up during the night to urinate.
- He is experiencing pain and cramps.
- He complains about pain in the lower back and in the groin.

A Small Gland with a Great Potential for Pain

The prostate gland is a small organ located at the junction of the urethra and the bladder. It produces a milky secretion, which, when ejaculated, is the medium in which the sperm can move. Without this secretion, the sperm wouldn't be able to travel toward a female ovum.

Whatever the changes in the prostate gland are, they have an immediate effect on the urethra and thus also on the ability to pass water. If, for example, the prostate becomes inflamed through either bacteria such as streptococci or through a urinary tract infection that hasn't prop-

Inflammation of the testes should be taken very seriously. Typical symptoms are swelling of one testicle, reddening, and severe pain. Sometimes these symptoms are accompanied by fever. If this condition isn't treated immediately with antibiotics (which can be effectively supported by enzymes), it could, if worse comes to worst, lead to sterility.

Plant Extracts against Prostate Problems
- Pumpkin seed oil, pumpkin seeds. Both are well suited for use in fresh green salads. Pumpkin seeds can also be eaten as a snack, just like peanuts.
- Extract from the roots of stinging nettle
- Goldenrod extract
- Horsetail extract
- Birch leaf extract

You can blend these four healing herbs or use them individually to prepare a tea. For this, measure out 1 teaspoon per cup and add to boiling water. Infuse for approximately 10 minutes. Drink three cups of the infusion per day.

Plant extracts combined with vitamin E are also very beneficial.

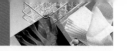

erly healed, this can result in swelling, which in turn causes the urethra to narrow. The result is a constant urge to pass water, and pain when doing so. Poor urine flow that is reduced to dripping indicates that the urethra has been affected as well. There is a possibility that the prostate may even expand in the other direction, affecting the bowels and thus bowel movements.

Prostate Tumors

It has been established that men, too, go through a change similar to menopause. The male hormones are reduced in favor of the female hormones. But this happens only to a certain degree—a man's fertility is retained completely. Prostate tumors, which are usually benign, can occur as a result of these hormonal changes.

This growth in the prostate can be of varying size. Because of it, passing water becomes such a serious problem that a small amount of urine remains in the bladder every time, creating an excellent medium in which all kinds of bacteria can thrive. Should the condition become acute, the patient will have no control over bladder function at all and urine will drip uncontrollably.

How the Doctor Can Help

In the case of prostate complaints, a visit to the doctor is crucial and should take place without delay. If the prostate is enlarged because of a tumor, plant-based medications can achieve a great deal if they are used early on. If they don't help, or if the tumor is already quite large, the doctor may prescribe female hormones. As a last resort and toughest measure, radiation therapy or surgery can be used to remove the tumor.

Enzymes Accelerate the Healing Process

In the case of prostatitis (inflammation of the prostate gland) caused by bacteria, enzymes come into their own with their two strengths: fighting inflammation and reducing swelling. With enzymes, the problems and the pain when urinating will disappear rapidly. However, bear in mind that, in most cases, enzymes alone won't help. A bac-

Tip
It is understandable that men don't like to talk about prostate complaints, either to their doctor or their wife or partner. But the longer the treatment of this condition is delayed, the more serious it becomes. Should you notice the symptoms of a possible prostate problem, try to broach the subject gently.

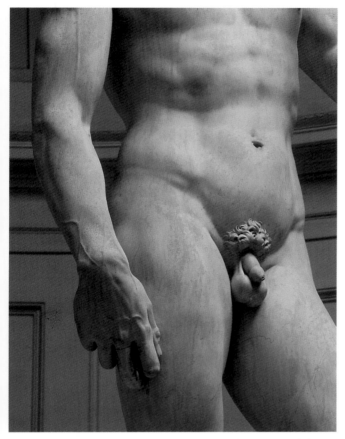

Once hormonal changes have caused the enlargement of the prostate gland, it usually takes some time before the first real problems occur.

Infections of the urinary tract can affect men of all ages. The causes are the same as for women: infection, usually caused by bacteria. Not changing out of wet swimwear and suffering a chill is just as harmful for men as it is for women. Men also shouldn't underestimate the risk of contracting an infection through sexual intercourse. And remember, both partners always need to be treated if one of them has a urinary tract infection.

terial inflammation of the prostate gland should always be treated with antibiotics as well. Sometimes a chronic inflammation of the prostate develops, often without symptoms and evidence of bacteria. In this case, antibiotics have no effect and therefore are no longer necessary.

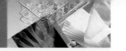

Inflammation of the Prostate without Bacteria
There is a type of inflammation of the prostate gland in which bacteria do not have a part. Medical science calls this "abacterial prostatitis." This is caused by pathogens against which antibiotics have no power. The treatment of this condition is far more time-consuming and can last up to six months. Even the doctor can't prescribe anything other than painkillers, antispasmodic medicines, and hip baths—unless he or she prescribes enzyme preparations, in which case the patient's suffering could be over in only six weeks.

A medical study of men with abacterial prostatitis revealed that 45 percent of the men were healed after a six-week course of enzymes, and, in 30 percent, the symptoms had decreased.

Enzymes to Help You Stay Young and Beautiful Longer

Enzymes are not the ultimate fountain of youth, nor do they work miracles against wrinkles. But if you take a closer look at the way they work inside the body, you will see that they can make a valuable contribution toward maintaining youthfulness and beauty.

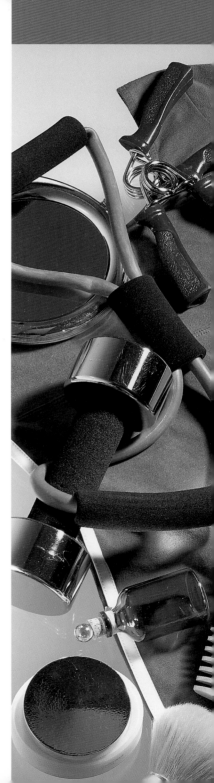

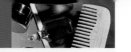

Staying Healthy and Dynamic as You Grow Older

What are the factors that cause aging? Is the aging process preprogrammed genetically? Do our organs, our metabolism, and other body functions simply become sluggish over the years? Or does the process start in the mind? Worldwide, the research into geriatrics is running at full speed in order to understand the aging process. However, many facts are already known today.

Enzymes for a Longer Life

According to our genetic programming, there seems to be no reason why we shouldn't all live to 110 or 120 years of age. And, in reality, we are coming closer and closer to this ideal. In highly industrialized countries, average life expectancy for women today is around age 80 and for men approximately 78 years of age.

The Sum of All Vices

It is true that many people these days live to a ripe old age, but most of them don't enter old age active and able-bodied with unspoiled enthusiasm. Once they have retired and should be enjoying the world around them, most people are struggling with serious illnesses. The quality of their lives and their capabilities are severely hampered by a number of ailments.

Unfortunately, many people have only themselves to blame. Many age-related complaints, such as a disturbed stomach and bowel function, a sluggish metabolism, and heart and circulatory problems, are the result of all the "sins against health" committed over a lifetime. The main "sins" are a poor diet, obesity, and too much alcohol, caffeine, and nicotine, as well as stress and a lack of exercise. There are other factors that we can't influence as much, like environmental poisons and diseases that run in the family.

> "Premature aging with all its consequences is mainly the result of enzyme deficiencies."
> —Max Wolf, founder of systemic enzyme therapy

100

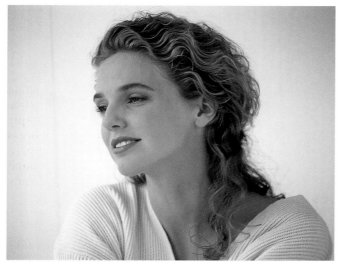

Enzymes ensure that the skin remains firm and supple, and they protect against premature wrinkles.

Nevertheless, leading a health-conscious life could at least help in part to guard against them.

Cells—Life's Building Blocks

All rejuvenation and renewal of the body takes place in its individual cells. As long as they continue to divide and renew themselves, all is well. But there are limits to these processes. And not all cells of the body have the same potential for dividing. The genetic program of each and every one of the 60 trillion cells in our bodies determines how often a cell will divide in a lifetime. Red blood cells, which transport the oxygen needed for life, divide every four months, and the cells of the intestinal walls divide every few days. Liver cells can divide up to 80 times during the course of a person's life.

All cells therefore divide and renew themselves at a certain rate. The genetic code of a cell also contains information about the maximum age a person can reach, provided

There are many secrets having to do with aging that geriatric science has not yet been able to uncover. It is, however, obvious that enzymes can exert a positive influence on some aging processes, as they encourage cell renewal, prevent arteriosclerosis, and support the oxygen supply of the body.

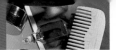

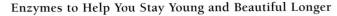

Premature Wear and Tear

In some people, the first warning signs of premature aging due to an unhealthy lifestyle manifest as early as age 40:

- In many, the digestive system no longer functions properly.
- The first heart problems appear.
- Vein complaints indicate circulatory problems.
- Depression, disturbed sleep, and a lack of concentration mean that the soul is suffering, and that opens the door to many psychosomatic illnesses.
- Increased susceptibility to infections indicates a weakened immune system.
- Wrinkles appear prematurely, as the connective tissue is no longer supple and elastic.
- Muscles and joints show the first signs of wear and tear, if for no other reason than that they haven't been exercised sufficiently for many years.
- The body's oxygen supply is poor, because blood circulation and respiration are disturbed.

According to current research, you can exert a significant influence on your quality of life in old age with a healthy diet, exercise, and a stable frame of mind, as well as with enzymes and coenzymes.

the circumstances are right and the person doesn't die prematurely as the result of an accident or a disease.

When Nature Shifts Down a Gear

Unfortunately, cell division does not go on forever. Over the years, the process gradually slows down, which means that the aging body has to be careful not to overexert itself. Nature still guards the secret of what the genetic program of cell division is like, but one thing is certain: Enzymes play an important role in this process.

Nothing Operates without Enzymes

A cell is viable only if it receives sufficient amounts of oxygen and nutrients. Enzymes ensure a trouble-free absorption of oxygen and nutrients in the metabolism of each individual cell, allowing the cells to remain fully functional longer. Try to move around and exercise as much as possible. This improves your overall metabolism and, with it,

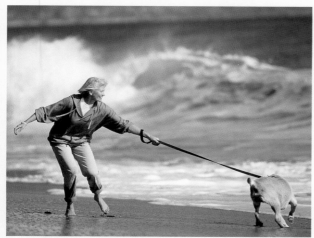

Active enzymes will keep you fit into old age.

Enzymes for the Best Years of Your Life

As you grow older, high enzyme levels can be very beneficial, regardless of whether the enzymes are produced by the
body itself or supplemented by taking enzyme preparations.
Enzymes accomplish the following:

- They ensure that cell renewal happens more efficiently
  and takes place longer.
- They support the cells of the connective tissue, maintain-
  ing firmer skin.
- They help to prevent arteriosclerosis.
- They protect the heart by promoting blood circulation.
- They improve the oxygen supply to all organs.
- They strengthen the body's defenses and protect the body
  from infections.
- They remove dead cells and their waste products before
  they can do any harm.
- They help to make existing age-related complaints more
  bearable or even may heal them.
- They improve the digestive system.
- They keep the metabolism up to speed.

Recent research
indicates that enzymes,
if administered over
many years, may
possibly protect one
from Alzheimer's
disease. Enzymes can
delay the onset of this
dreaded condition and
seem to ensure that the
accompanying relentless
loss of memory
progresses less rapidly.

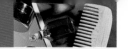
your enzyme balance. In addition, make sure that you eat a varied diet with plenty of raw fruit and vegetables and whole-grain products, all of which contain large amounts of coenzymes. In this way, your enzymes will retain their full power.

Cell Structure

The outside of the cell, its protective layer, is called the cell membrane or the cell wall. It protects the inside of the cell from pathogens and other harmful influences. It also fulfills an important function in the body's metabolism. The cell surface isn't smooth, but covered with receptors. These

Aging is not a disease. Hardly anyone in the industrialized world these days dies of old age. If we succeeded in defeating heart disease and cancer, we would probably be able to reach our biologically programmed age of 115 years.

One look into a cell shows that the nucleus of each cell produces its own special enzymes that control the numerous tasks of the cell.

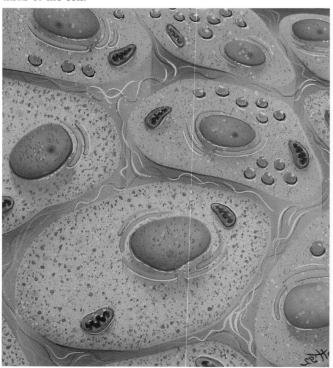

receptors absorb the nutrients as well as hormones and other substances that the cell requires.

The cell membrane also houses a kind of communication system that enables cells to exchange messages. Here are two examples of how this works: If one cell dies as a result of high alcohol levels, the neighboring cell can alert others to divide in order to replace the lost cell. If a virus threatens to enter a cell, the cell can use the communication system to call for help and even state which weapons are needed to defeat the enemy.

The Heart of the Cell

At the center of each cell is its most important component, the nucleus. It contains important genetic information and initiates cell division. In cell division, the nucleus divides in two, with each new nucleus carrying identical genetic information in its chromosomes.

The most important life-sustaining process in a cell is its respiration, which actually refers to the entire process of nutrient absorption, which in a cell takes place with the help of oxygen. Oxygen converts nutrients into energy. The most important suppliers of nutrients are sugars (glucose and fructose), protein, which the digestive enzymes split up into individual amino acids, and fat, which is converted into fatty acids. How the resulting energy is used depends on which task a cell fulfills in the body. Brain cells, for example, use energy for thought processes, coordinating physical processes in the body, and giving commands. Nerve cells transmit messages, and muscle cells move.

Enzymes Are Always Present

Enzymes participate in all processes linked to cell metabolism—that is, the supply and absorption of nutrients and the control of cell respiration. Those enzymes that are part of the vital process of energy production in a cell are without a doubt the most important enzymes in the body. They are located within the cell's power generators, the mitochondria, and from there send out the impulses necessary to control respiration.

Enzymes ensure that oxygen attaches itself to hemoglobin in a fraction of a second and, at its destination, is transported into the cells just as quickly. This process needs to be fully functional in old age as well.

105

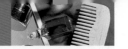

Essential: Coenzymes

In this context, the previously mentioned coenzymes are of great importance too. For the respiratory chain, niacin (vitamin B3) and its related coenzyme NAD play a significant role. The coenzyme FAD, which is formed from vitamin B2, is needed by the cell for the conversion of nutrients into energy. Combined, they all enable enzymes to do their work in the respiratory chain.

Older people, in particular, should have at least two glasses of this drink per day (diluted with mineral water, if

---

A Coenzyme Drink

1. Mix the three juices in a glass. Add the oat bran, stirring until it has dissolved completely.
2. Add dried coconut to taste, and garnish with pieces of fruit. Drink immediately to prevent the coenzymes from being destroyed through exposure to the air.

Ingredients for two large glasses: 6½ oz. (200 ml) orange juice, 3½ oz. (100 ml) carrot juice, 6½ oz. (200 ml) mango juice, 1 tablespoon instant oat bran, dried coconut, and pieces of fruit to garnish

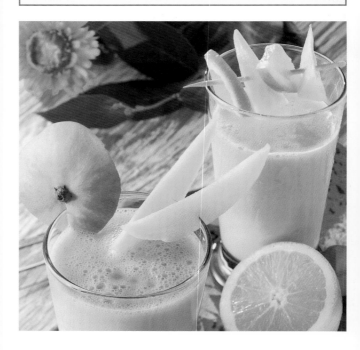

desired). Apart from the coenzymes, it ensures the intake of important minerals and plenty of fluid.

Beneficial in Old Age: Coenzyme Q10

A miracle drug for heart complaints—this is how the press extolled the discovery of Q10, a substance similar to a vitamin that can be found in many foods. However, as with almost everything in medicine, this coenzyme has nothing to do with miracles. Q10 has been found to be an important coenzyme for those enzymes that participate in the energy metabolism of cells. Present research has also shown that that this coenzyme seems to play an important role when it comes to the heart.

With advancing age, a weak heart is a common problem and is usually the result of premature wear. A comparison of healthy heart tissue with a weakened heart muscle showed interesting results: The diseased heart displayed a severe Q10 deficiency in contrast to the healthy heart. A further examination of the blood of patients with heart disease showed the same Q10 deficiencies.

Q10 Keeps Your Heart Young

Enzyme research has discovered that the cells of the heart contain a large number of enzymes important for respiration, and that these enzymes require the coenzyme Q10. Without Q10, the enzymes of the respiratory chain of the heart muscle cells are practically paralyzed. It is therefore not surprising that older people with a deficiency of this coenzyme develop heart problems.

When older patients were given regular Q10 supplements with their food, the performance of their hearts improved considerably and surprisingly quickly. A few weeks was all it took, and without any additional medication.

Numerous studies into Q10 have been conducted in Japan, the United States, and Europe. As early as 1989, a group of research scientists was able to prove that the decrease of Q10 levels in the body is definitely age-dependent.

An important word of warning: If you suffer from high blood pressure, it would be a mistake to discontinue your usual medication and take Q10 instead. It is imperative that you consult your doctor first.

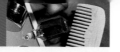
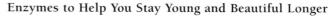
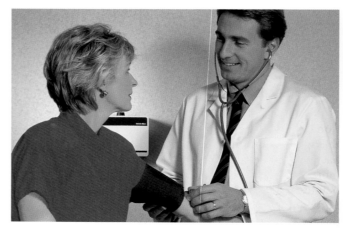

High blood pressure has few symptoms. It is therefore advisable to have your blood pressure checked regularly.

Tip
The coenzyme Q10 is contained in food such as meat, fish, poultry, and eggs. Current findings, however, suggest that the amounts normally taken with food are no longer sufficient in old age.

A New Weapon against High Blood Pressure

Many people start to suffer from dangerously high blood pressure when they are middle-aged. This condition can become life-threatening with time, as it puts too much strain on the heart, causing it to continuously work harder. The patient may possibly not notice for a long time that anything is amiss. Apart from organic causes, permanently high blood pressure is brought on by a lack of exercise, excess weight, nicotine, and alcohol.

In cases of high blood pressure, the delicate balance between the streaming pressure of the blood and the tension of the vascular walls is severely disturbed. The vascular walls are under immense strain, and this results in more frequent minuscule injuries to which blood platelets can stick and over time develop into larger deposits. If this development remains untreated, it can cause a stroke, clogging of the coronary arteries, angina pectoris (a painful sensation in the chest), and a chronically weak heart. Yet impressive research from the United States, Japan, and Italy has proven that, by solely supplementing the diet with Q10, blood pressure can be effectively lowered in the early and middle stages.

Remaining Fit and Active into Old Age

Enzymes are an important part of the immune system; all of the natural defense and self-healing mechanisms function fully only if enzymes are present. Enzymes stimulate the immune system especially in the fight against viruses, bacteria, cell waste, chemicals, and other toxins. The more enzyme levels are reduced in old age, the more helpless a person is when faced with the onslaught of numerous germs and environmental poisons as well as the strain caused by metabolic waste products.

Enzymes Also Age

As with all other body functions, enzyme activity declines with increasing age. Fewer enzymes are available, and, to make matters worse, the remaining enzymes no longer work as fast as they used to. The entire aging process, however, hinges on the body's immune system, because not only does it fight germs but it also initiates important self-healing processes. But if a lack of enzymes and other biological substances impede the immune system in its work, a vicious cycle is set in motion.

Enzyme Deficiencies Paralyze Metabolism

With a lack of enzymes, metabolic waste and toxins are no longer transported away fast enough and in sufficient quantities. Instead, they accumulate in the body's tissues and fluids. Metabolic functions like digestion and blood circulation can suffer long-term damage as a result of excessive strain, as can many organs, such as the liver and the kidneys. On the one hand, these harmful processes in the metabolism impair the work of the macrophages, making it easier for germs to find a foothold in the body. On the other hand, they pave the way for chronic conditions due to wear and for autoimmune diseases. However, you can exert some influence on how soon and to what extent such physical decline in old age begins.

It is a good idea for older people to undergo enzyme treatment at regular intervals. But this doesn't mean that they shouldn't actively look after their health anymore.

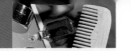

How to Support Your Enzymes and Your Immune System

- Try to get plenty of sleep. Most people need about eight hours of sleep a night. It is best if you can go to sleep at the same time each night.
- Enjoy alcohol only in moderation, and refrain from nicotine completely.
- Try to get adequate and regular exercise in the open air. Aim for a one-hour walk per week.
- Eat a healthy diet with lots of fruit, vegetables, and whole-grain products. Drink at least 2 quarts, or liters, of fluids a day.
- Use Kneipp's water therapies, for example, in the shower every morning. Try to go to a sauna once a month.

Be honest: Do you smoke? Is your life too stressful? Do you have a poor diet? Discover your areas of weakness, and write down how you intend to overcome them and by when. Jotting down these intentions in a diary can serve as a helpful reminder.

Red Alert for Your Immune System

It would be a mistake to think that the deterioration of your immune system doesn't start until you are 50 or 60 years of age. Depending on your lifestyle and on your health, it may be advisable to start strengthening your

How Strong Are Your Body's Defenses?

If you can answer yes to several of the questions below, you should read the next few pages very carefully, because your immune system probably needs a boost.

- Do you catch every flu virus that goes around, and are you very susceptible to other infections as well?
- Do you constantly feel tired, sluggish, and as if you aren't realizing your capabilities?
- Do you frequently suffer from headaches, bloodshot eyes, or a lack of concentration, for no apparent reason?
- Do you take longer than other people to recover from an illness?
- Do you frequently suffer relapses after an illness?
- Are you under enormous psychological strain—for example, from stress at work or problems in a relationship?

immune system when you are as young as age 30. Use the checklist below to determine how strong your body's defenses currently are.

Boosting Your Immune System the Easy Way—with Water

The cold-water treatments devised by Pastor Kneipp (1821 to 1897) from Germany activate in the metabolism all those enzymes and other biological substances that support the immune system. The treatments described below can easily be carried out at home.

Hot-and-Cold Showers

Alternating hot-and-cold showers are best taken first thing in the morning. Start by showering for a few minutes with

Alternating hot-and-cold showers awaken your immune system and your enzymes. This is ideal if you have low blood pressure or tend to be tired and grumpy in the morning.

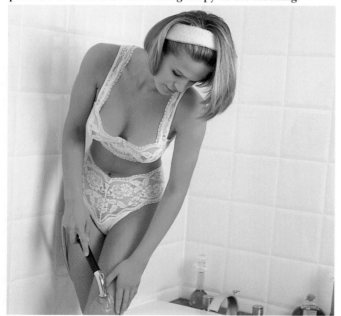

Tip
If you can cope with the heat of a sauna, then you should go to one regularly. The contrast between the extremely dry heat of the sauna and the cold water that you pour over yourself promotes the removal of toxins from the body and improves circulation and metabolism. This in turn will activate enzymes and other biocatalysts.

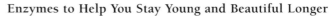

hot water (about 104 degrees Fahrenheit, or 40 degrees Celsius). Then shower with cold water for a few seconds, followed by another three or four minutes of hot water. Repeat this process several times. Even hot-and-cold showers for your arms and legs alone will stimulate your circulation. Always finish with a hot shower, and don't dry yourself off afterward.

Paddling

Paddling is a great way to boost your immune system. Run cold water in your bath up to about mid-calf height. Carefully walk up and down in your bath for several minutes, making sure to raise your feet above the water level with every step. It's helpful to do this paddling treatment just before bedtime, because, according to Pastor Kneipp, it will also help you get a good night's sleep.

The body's self-healing powers are still the best weapons we have against disease. Doctors from all branches of medicine are united for once on this point. Therefore, researchers have been concentrating on substances that are able to significantly improve the body's self-healing powers. The results thus far have shown that enzymes are one of the most powerful weapons we have to influence the self-healing process.

When pouring water over your arms, run the water over the entire length of your arm, top to bottom.

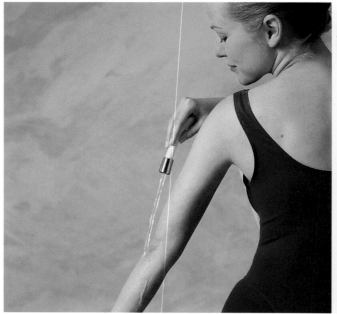

Arm and Leg Treatment

This treatment focuses on the arms and/or the legs. First, gently pour pleasantly warm water over your arms or legs. Follow this with a quick cold shower. Then repeat the warm water on your arms or legs. Carry out this process several times.

Stress—the Immune System's Greatest Enemy

Hans Selye, the founder of modern stress research, distinguishes between two forms of stress. On the one hand, there is positive stress, which is stimulating and allows people to use their abilities to the fullest. Negative stress, on the other hand, is always experienced as a strain and exerts too much pressure on the individual.

When we talk about stress today, we are usually referring to the negative type. In this context, stress is synonymous with pressure, strain, and tension. It is no wonder that constant stress can cause illness, as it maintains a permanent but entirely unnecessary state of alert. As a result,

Tip
After a stressful day, lie down quietly for a few minutes, loosen any restrictive clothing, and try not to think about your problems for a while. Instead, visualize something pleasant that you enjoy—for example, a summer meadow splashed with flowers or a secluded beach at sunset.

Stress can have many causes: too much work, relationship problems, or perhaps just a traffic jam during rush hour.

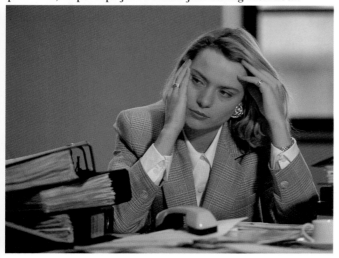

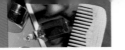

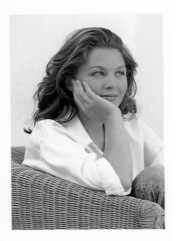

**Relaxation will restore
your enzyme balance.**

Twelve Ways to Conquer Stress

- Draw up a plan for the day, allowing for regular meals and breaks.
- Make a list of your problems and unresolved issues, and tackle them one after the other.
- Speak to friends about your problems.
- Gradually remove excessive strain from your life.
- Never just swallow your anger, but state clearly if you disagree with something and why.
- Rid yourself of feelings of guilt and a bad conscience.
- Improve your feeling of self-worth by identifying at least 20 positive characteristics that apply to you and writing them down on paper.
- Learn tried-and-tested relaxation techniques, such as visualizations, yoga, tai chi, and meditation.
- Avoid alcohol, caffeine, and nicotine.
- If you are nervous or can't sleep, choose plant-based remedies (valerian, hops, melissa) over strong conventional medications.
- Why not have a laugh at your own expense once in a while?
- Most importantly, learn to say NO!

---

the immune system and its enzymes also constantly work overtime, wasting valuable energy. Stress is harmful for the entire body, because it paralyzes vital processes, particularly immune reactions and enzyme activity. In addition, such chronic, excessive strain on the psyche encourages all kinds of dependency and drug abuse, and is the greatest cause of all psychosomatic illnesses.

Fitness—the Magic Word

One thing is for certain: If you are fit, you will remain physically and mentally agile for longer, and your heart, circulation, respiration, and metabolism will benefit as well. You will also maintain your level of performance, continue to enjoy life, and stay mentally stable and balanced. In addi-

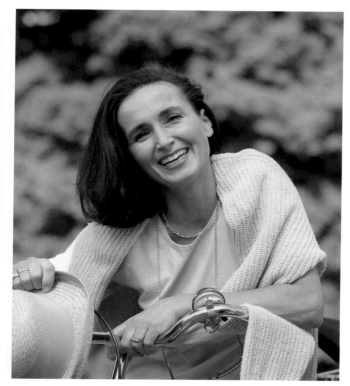

Riding a bike is ideal for someone not used to exercise.

Tip
Mineral drinks and fresh fruit are perfect snacks for athletic people, because they supply their own enzymes (activated by the exercise) with important coenzymes.

tion, being fit is great for your body: Your muscles, joints, ligaments, and tendons will stay flexible, and even the little gray cells benefit from the smallest amount of physical exercise. A short walk, for example, increases circulation in the cerebrum. This means that more enzymes reach the cerebrum and initiate numerous chemical reactions, which in turn have a very beneficial effect on your overall well-being, concentration, and entire body.

Keep Fit for Your Enzymes' Sake

But what do exercise and physical fitness have to do with enzymes? It's simple: With every movement you make, you activate many thousands of little processes in your body,

115

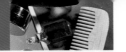

initiate innumerable biochemical reactions, and encourage the production of many of your own enzymes, which will improve your health, give you a greater overall sense of joy in living, and increase your ability to cope with stress.

Exercise—Don't Become Rusty

A 60-year-old woman who has never exercised in her life has, over the years, lost between 20 and 25 percent of her original capabilities. Accordingly, her enzymes will be fairly sluggish. Men can even lose up to a third of their capabilities. If you decide at age 60 to go for it and start exercising, then you will be able, after only 10 to 12 weeks, to achieve the same level of fitness of someone who is 20 years younger!

About 70 percent of our health and life expectancy are determined by genetic factors. The remaining 30 percent, however, are in our own hands.

Don't force your body to its limits, especially when you are older. You should still be able to talk to someone while you are exercising.

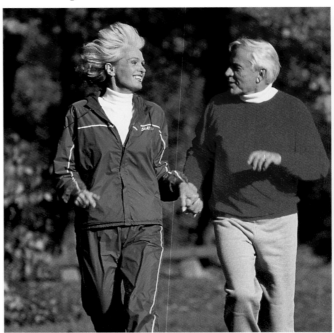

Test Your Fitness
In 30 seconds, you should manage:

	Sit-ups	Push-ups	Squats
Age 20–30			
Women	18	19	26
Men	23	24	30
Age 30–40			
Women	15	18	24
Men	20	19	28
Age 40–50			
Women	12	16	20
Men	15	16	24
Over age 50 (only after having consulted your doctor)			
Women	10	15	15
Men	12	14	18

As a general rule, the earlier you start exercising regularly, the longer you will stay young. At age 60, you can still be just as fit as a 40-year-old. A well-known German medical scientist once said about the problem of reduced performance is that at birth we are fit for life, and that we lose this fitness only because of the lack of exercise that rules our lives.

Have Fun!
Exercise has the following health benefits: endurance, strength, coordination, agility, and speed. For amateurs, speed is the least important. Your health will benefit mainly from endurance, strength, and agility.

However, when choosing the type of exercise that is best for you, the above criteria aren't the only things that are important. Experts agree that psychological factors should also be considered. You should choose a form of exercise that you enjoy doing. Therefore, think about whether you like to exercise alone, by jogging in the fresh air, for example, or if you prefer competitive sports, such as tennis. In addition, bear in mind whether or not you have any med-

Tip
Headaches, a lack of concentration, signs of fatigue, forgetfulness—all may point to the beginning of a mental decline. But if you want to maintain an active mind and active enzymes, especially those that supply the cells with carbohydrates and oxygen, exercise your body in the open air and regularly exercise your mind as well.

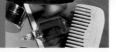

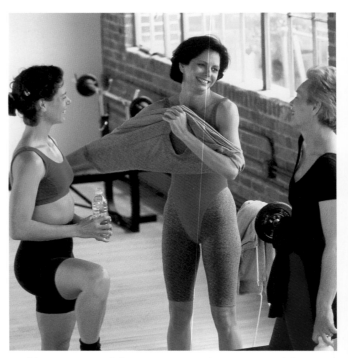

Building up strength by exercising at the gym is good for women of all ages, because it keeps the muscles and the bones active.

Tip
The body benefits most from the so-called endurance sports, such as walking, swimming, cycling, and cross-country skiing.

ical condition that might rule out a particular sport. If in doubt, consult your doctor.

Exercising at the Gym
Building up your strength at the gym can be very helpful, especially if you have only started exercising at age 40 or older. By that time, you will have lost approximately 20 to 40 percent of your muscle (replaced by fat!). Building up your strength means rebuilding your muscles and regulating vital metabolic processes. In addition, if it is done correctly, this type of exercise will help to prevent damage caused by poor posture. The only drawback is that you are not exercising in the open air.

Cycling

Cycling is an excellent sport to improve endurance, while also being relatively easy on the joints and the bones. Cycling stimulates the heart and circulation, and it increases lung capacity and therefore oxygen intake. After a tour of cycling, your metabolism will run at a higher rate for up to 24 hours, and you will definitely feel all the better for it. Also, with bike riding, there is the additional factor of mental relaxation when you ride through beautiful countryside.

Tennis

Tennis is not especially beneficial for the heart and circulation, and it puts the muscles and the tendons under a great deal of stress rather than improving them. However, tennis is good for the metabolism, if only because of the fact that you are exercising outdoors. It is advisable, however, to practice an endurance sport, in addition to tennis, such as walking, cycling, or swimming.

Swimming

Like all other endurance sports, swimming stimulates the heart, circulation, and respiration, and activates those enzymes that are responsible for the oxygen transport in the blood. This means a lasting improvement in the oxygen supply to the whole body. Because the muscles and the joints are moved gently, swimming is just about the ideal sport for people whose bodies display the first signs of wear.

Walking and Jogging

Brisk walking and moderate jogging are also ideal for the heart, circulation, respiration, and muscles. In addition, they are terrific outlets for stress and anger, so the mind and the nerves benefit equally. With these forms of exercise, it is essential not to overdo it and to have the correct footwear.

Squash may exercise your ability to react, but it puts a strain on the bones and the ligaments. It also bears a high risk of injury, particularly for beginners. But if you like this fast sport, you should think about taking enzymes as a preventive measure.

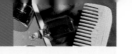

Eating Your Way to a Younger You

Make sure you get an adequate intake of coenzymes—that is, vitamins, minerals, and trace elements—in your diet. With a sufficient supply of coenzymes, your overall metabolism will improve, you will develop a slimmer and trimmer figure, and the circulation of your skin will be improved, giving you a rosy complexion. By eating a diet with plenty of coenzymes, you will become healthier and look younger and more beautiful!

Healthy Cooking

In your younger years, your diet isn't all that critical, but once you've reached 30 years of age, when your body's enzyme production slows down and your metabolism has already suffered some damage, the first consequences of an unhealthy diet may become apparent. But don't despair—even if you are older than age 40, you can still repair a lot of the damage by switching to a healthier, more sensible diet. The important rule of thumb for a long and healthy life is, the older you are, the more attention you should pay to a healthy, high-quality diet with plenty of nutrients. Dietary sins should only be the exception, not the rule.

Nutrient Density—the Formula for a Slimmer Figure

Counting calories rarely leads to a good figure and a healthy body. The important factor in everything that we eat is nutrient density. This refers to the relationship of high-calorie fats, carbohydrates, and proteins to nutrients like vitamins, minerals, and trace elements. As a general rule, half of our caloric intake should come from carbohydrates, 35 percent should come from fat, and 15 percent should come from proteins. The German nutritional expert Professor Michael Hamm has compiled a list of eight nutrient groups that our bodies need every day (see the table on page 123).

In light of the new concept of nutrient density, refined white sugar doesn't get the thumbs up, as it only supplies one nutrient, sugar. This is a rather poor show in comparison to other suppliers of sugar like fruit that contain plenty of additional nutrients.

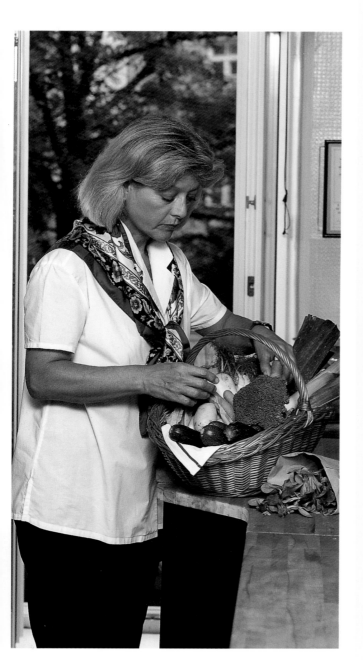

Tip
Fresh vegetables will help you to stay young and fit, because they contain numerous substances without which the body's own enzymes couldn't function.

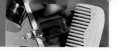

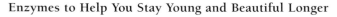

Nutrients are those substrates that enzymes need in order to produce energy and vitality. The better the quality of our food, the more our enzymes give back to us, in the form of power, endurance, ability to concentrate, health, and good looks.

What We Need to Live:

1. Carbohydrates, which the body converts into blood sugar (with the help of enzymes, of course), are the fastest suppliers of energy. Sugar itself, however, is a poor supplier of carbohydrates, as it can only raise blood-sugar levels for a short time. The table on the next page lists better carbohydrate sources.

2. Fiber is necessary as a lubricant for the bowels, ensuring regular, problem-free digestion.

3. Water is one of the most important nutrients. All cells need water to be able to grow and divide. Without water, blood, lymph, and the fluid in tissue would not be able to flow and therefore couldn't transport enzymes to their destinations. We also require water for our own cooling system—if we perspire a lot, we use about 5 quarts, or liters, of water a day.

4. Proteins are counted among the building blocks required by all cells for all life-sustaining processes in the body. The body uses them to produce its own enzymes. A protein deficiency (rare in most places in the Western world) could therefore lead to an enzyme deficiency. However, try to avoid butter, as it will only raise your cholesterol level, not to mention your weight.

5. Lipids (fats) are important sources of energy. Make sure that you eat the right kinds of fat, such as essential, polyunsaturated fatty acids from vegetable oils, high-quality margarine, and fish.

6. Vitamins have mainly a supporting function, such as in assisting enzymes. They also fulfill important tasks in the metabolism, especially for the nervous system, the brain, muscles, digestion, and the immune system.

7. Minerals also assist enzymes and other biological substances. In addition, they participate directly in many processes in the body (for example, magnesium is required for muscle function).

8. Trace elements are those minerals of which the body only requires traces. Nevertheless, deficiencies of selenium, iron, and iodine are quite common, hindering the proper use and absorption of many vitamins, carbohydrates, and fats.

Where to Find Nutrients

Nutrients	Foods
Carbohydrates	Bread, potatoes, whole-grain products, brown rice, vegetables, cereal products, pasta
Fiber	Bread, all whole-grain products, potatoes, legumes, vegetables, fruit
Water	All drinks, soups, fruit, vegetables
Protein	Soy products, fish, meat, dairy products, eggs, legumes
Fat (Lipids)	Cold-water fish such as herring, mackerel, cod, salmon, trout (especially for essential linoleic acid and alpha-linolenic acid), vegetable oils, fatty meat, sausages, cheese, nuts, seeds, butter, margarine
Vitamins	Fruit, vegetables, herbs, nuts, seeds, vegetable oils, rice, meat, fish, eggs
Minerals	Vegetables, fruit, lettuce, herbs, eggs, meat, fish, whole-grain products, milk, dairy products, nuts
Trace elements	Leafy green vegetables, wheat germ, sweetbreads, whole-grain products, fish and seafood (iodine), meat (selenium, zinc, iron), mushrooms, garlic (selenium), nuts, seeds, cheese

Tip
Enzymes only function in a team with their coenzymes. The same is true for all nutrients and the biological substances required for their absorption. Alone, the nutrients cannot achieve anything, but with their helpers they are invincible. Therefore, never go on a one-sided weight-loss diet—you can be sure that your body will be lacking important nutrients.

How to Eat Healthily

A varied diet made up of high-quality, fresh ingredients is best (fruit, vegetables, whole-grain products, fish, milk and dairy products, lean meat). Eat raw produce as often as possible. For instance, prepare a salad from grated vegetables—this way, you can be sure that you will preserve their vitamins, minerals, and trace elements. Bypass the deli

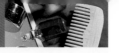

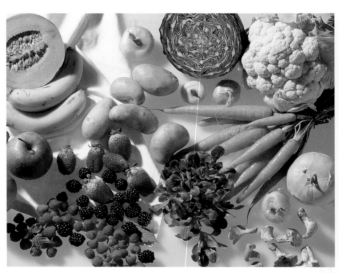

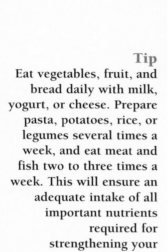

Tip
Eat vegetables, fruit, and bread daily with milk, yogurt, or cheese. Prepare pasta, potatoes, rice, or legumes several times a week, and eat meat and fish two to three times a week. This will ensure an adequate intake of all important nutrients required for strengthening your enzyme balance.

Fresh fruit and vegetables taste great and are good for you!

counter, and go easy on meat, especially if it isn't lean. Eat little sugar and baked goods made with white flour, because they contain hardly any important nutrients. Ensure a daily fluid intake of at least 2 quarts, or liters. Mineral water, herbal teas, and unsweetened fruit and vegetable juices are best. Of course, water can also be found in soups, fruit, and vegetables.

Try not to put too much strain on your body—even for healthy people, it is better to eat five small meals a day than three big meals. Our bodies need nutrients all day long, so it isn't sensible to supply them all in one meal. If your lifestyle requires you to eat a lot of fast food or cafeteria meals, you would be well advised to supplement your enzyme balance. Brewers' yeast is a good source of such coenzymes as the B vitamins, selenium, zinc, and manganese.

Enzymes as a Beauty Treatment

Ancient cultures such as that of Native Americans applied meat and certain plants to wounds to facilitate the healing process. They didn't know, however, that the healing was caused by enzymes. But this was soon discovered in the early stages of enzyme therapy, which included medicinal ointments for wounds as a classic treatment. It was later found that the skin could be improved with enzymes, and that enzyme cosmetics could be used to fight the premature aging and wrinkling of the skin from the outside.

Enzymes in Cosmetics

The cosmetics industry discovered enzymes only a few years ago. Progress has recently been made in the areas of skin aging and formation of wrinkles.

The Structure of Our Skin

On an average, our skin has a thickness of 1 millimeter, but this varies depending on which part of the body we are looking at. The skin is at its thinnest on the lips and around the eyes, and at its thickest on the soles of the feet. The fingertips are the most sensitive parts of the skin, and the skin on the stomach area is the strongest. Nevertheless, the structure of the skin is the same, regardless of its location. It consists of three layers with an innumerable quantity of cells, including blood-vessel cells, nerve cells, muscle cells, and sebaceous- and sweat-gland cells. Of course, enzymes are active in all layers of the skin. Without them, the metabolic processes of the skin wouldn't function.

The Epidermis

This is the top layer of the skin and the part we see. Sometimes called the "germ layer," it is important for our good looks, because it forms those important cells that take

The skin contributes to the body's oxygen supply to a limited extent. In comparison to the lungs, it can manage only about 1 percent of air intake.

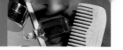

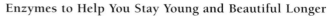

care of skin renewal. What we see are already dead, tiny keratin particles of these young cells.

Through washing and friction, we remove up to two billion of these skin particles daily, but they are replaced immediately from below. In this manner, the surface of the skin renews itself completely within a month. In addition to the immune cells, which we have already discussed, the epidermis plays host to those cells that are responsible for the frequently desired tan: the pigment cells. By producing the hormone melanin, they also provide some protection from UV rays.

Let's See What's under the Skin

The skin is one of the body's largest organs. It consists of three layers; the first two can be seen in the illustration below.

As long as our skin is intact, we don't notice most of its activities. But even when we sleep, it transmits sensory messages to other parts of the body, which then react accordingly. For example, the message "The body is cold" will trigger a reaction in the brain and cause us to get up and fetch another blanket.

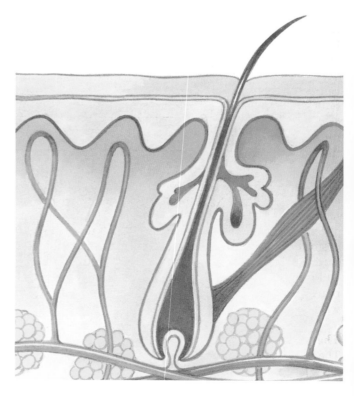

The Dermis

The dermis is the middle layer of the skin. It is here that important detoxifying processes take place. The dermis also serves as the water reservoir of the skin, as it contains collagenous fibers that can store a large amount of water, making the skin look fresh and firm. These water reservoirs are at their most efficient in young people; with increasing age, the cells of the collagenous fibers unfortunately become less elastic. Enzymes, however, are able to halt this process to a certain extent.

The dermis contains elastic fibers that enable the covering layer of our bodies to follow every movement without immediately displaying wrinkles or dents on the surface. In addition, the dermis contains numerous nerve fibers as well as the roots of sweat and sebaceous glands and hair follicles.

The blood circulation of the skin mainly takes place in the dermis as well. This is an important factor for youthful looks and a beautiful complexion. Numerous blood and lymph vessels traverse the dermis, transporting vital nutrients such as vitamins, minerals, proteins, and oxygen. These nutrients are needed by every single skin cell, but they would not reach their destination without enzymes. Waste products that cannot be secreted with sweat are transported away through the same vessels. If the exchange of vital nutrients and cell waste no longer works properly, the skin will bear testimony to this. As a result of poor blood circulation, it will become gray, with a parchment quality, and may display a tendency toward impurities.

Some of these problems can be partially remedied with cosmetics, as certain creams contain a lot of nutrients such as vitamins that improve enzyme activity in the skin. This will make the skin softer and more resilient. The collagenous fibers will be able to absorb more water, and minor wrinkles will disappear.

Many people make excessive use of deodorants, because they think that perspiration is always accompanied by an offensive odor. However, this is not true. The secreted sweat only develops an unpleasant smell if it comes into contact with bacteria living on the surface of the skin. The sweat secreted under the arms and in the genital area has a particularly unpleasant smell, because those parts of the body also have their own natural scent glands.

The Subcutis

The subcutis is the deeper layer of the dermis. It is the layer that causes problems for anyone who discovers, after

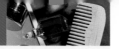

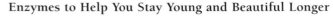

The Three Skin Types

- Normal skin has a rosy shimmer, looks slightly moist, and feels firm to the touch. The skin pores are barely visible.
- Dry skin feels rough and has no luster; instead, it has a parchment quality. It tends to develop red spots and can feel tight.
- Greasy skin looks oily and glistening, its pores are very enlarged, and it tends to become inflamed and develop pimples and blackheads. The complexion is pale and gray.

Free radicals play a significant role in the aging process and in many disorders of the skin. Yet enzymes, teamed up with their coenzymes, can help to forestall signs of aging and prevent certain skin conditions.

losing weight, that his or her skin looks wrinkly, saggy, and without luster.

Together with our friendly helpers, the enzymes, nature has built its energy deposits for emergencies right here in the subcutis. In other words, this is where the fat cells are. The subcutis itself is rather heavy, compared to the other skin layers, accounting for two-thirds of the total weight of the skin.

If we sometimes refer to chubby individuals as being "well padded," there is a reason for that. The fat stores in the subcutis have another important function: They also serve as protective padding for some of the internal organs, such as the liver and the kidneys, as well as for the muscles and the nerves.

The Function of Enzymes in the Skin

Few people in the Western world seem to appreciate the fact that our bodies build up stores in case times become harder. These layers of fat can be found in the subcutaneous tissue. Digestive enzymes help to store anything that isn't converted into energy immediately. In addition to fat, essential minerals and other nutrients are stored in the subcutis.

Glands in the Skin Excrete Toxins

Enzymes also participate actively in another important task that the skin fulfills: They help to transport away toxins

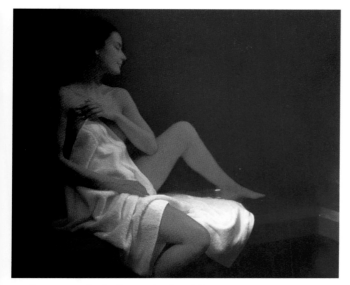

In the sauna, the body can be freed from toxins and waste products.

and waste products, which aren't just secreted by the kidneys but also through numerous sweat glands in the skin. Most of them are concentrated in the armpits, the palms of the hands, the soles of the feet, and the genital area.

The sweat glands are located deep down in the dermis, and sweat is secreted through tiny vessels onto the skin surface. It is not advisable to suppress the natural, detoxifying process of sweating with medication or through exaggerated hygiene. Sweating is a vital process! Under normal circumstances, every day we secrete about a quart, or liter, of sweat, made up of 99.5 percent water, as well as mineral salts, urea, fatty acids, and amino acids. If we exercise or work hard physically or if the weather is hot, we secrete more. There is good reason why doctors from different branches of medicine often advise us to "sweat it out," so that toxins and waste products are flushed out of the body.

Tip
Through sweating, the body loses a relatively high amount of potassium. You should therefore drink potassium-rich mineral water or, even better, a fruit-juice spritzer made up of one-third fruit juice and two-thirds sparkling mineral water.

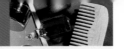

The First Barrier of the Immune System

Recent studies have found that the skin has its own immune system that saves the body's internal immune system a great deal of work. From this discovery, a new branch of science has developed: immune dermatology. It has found that the skin's immune system is activated by the thymus gland, which is located behind the sternum and sends its own messages. Enzymes also play a role in the skin's immune system, and you can give these enzymes effective support with a diet rich in coenzymes and possibly also with vitamins and enzymes in your cosmetics.

The Skin's Protective Layer

Battles on the skin surface take place exclusively in the skin's protective layer—which is the best reason to always take good care of your skin. This top layer of skin contains certain protein molecules (immunoglobulins) that, in conjunction with other substances (enzymes included, of course!), make up a perfectly formed defensive line. Whatever gets past them encounters the next barrier of the skin's immune system. The epidermis contains skin macrophages, which receive support from the keratinocytes, found between the epidermis and the dermis. They will devour each and every attacker, but only if the attacker gets too close.

As a rule, these defense cells are rather lazy and prefer to leave the hard work to others—namely, the skin patrol, made up of white blood cells, which are in a constant state of alert and ready for action. Just as in the immune system, they are informed by the skin macrophages about the enemy's location, numbers, and weapons. They will then immediately march off, using all their available strength.

The Enemy Doesn't Sleep

One would think that such a well-equipped defensive system could disarm any attacker, and that the body's immune system would therefore have much less work to do. But this is not the case, for two reasons. First of all, the enemy, whether a virus, a bacterium, or a fungus, is also well equipped. In order to outsmart the immune system, it con-

The protective outer layer of our skin has a great deal to endure. The American Health Foundation found that the skin has to withstand as many as 20,000 attacks a day from a variety of harmful substances.

130

The Skin's Protective Layer

The right pH level for the skin is 5.5—but what does this actually mean?

- The pH level is the unit of measurement for the amino acids on the skin surface that are contained in the natural layer of water and fat directly on the skin. This layer is made up of sebum, sweat, and cell particles of dead skin.
- The acid content of this protective film can vary considerably. It is measured on a scale of zero to 14. Levels up to six are considered acidic and ideal for the defense function of the skin. Seven is considered neutral. Levels of eight and above are considered alkaline and, with respect to the skin's defense function, extremely unhealthy.
- In addition to its defensive function, the protective layer of the skin works as a highly efficient barrier against dirt and controls the moisture content of the topmost skin layer.

Normal, healthy skin regenerates within an hour after washing with water and soap. The fat and moisture contents stabilize, and the acid level normalizes. The drier and more sensitive the skin is, however, the more it will be damaged by soap, shampoo, and dish-washing detergent. The typical symptoms of a damaged protective layer are reddening, itching, and rough and broken skin.

stantly comes up with new strategies and new types of camouflage. Secondly, the amount of harmful substances our bodies are subjected to has increased considerably in the recent past, whereas the number of defense cells remains the same. This means that the same number of defense troops has to cope with an ever-increasing number of enemy forces. It is therefore in our health's best interest to look after the protective layer of our skin.

The skin has two main enemies: water and soap. Someone who practices excessive hygiene and showers two to three times daily or takes frequent and long baths will wash away part of the skin's natural protective layer. The damage is even greater if you use soap to wash your skin. It is advisable, for this reason and especially if you have dry or sensitive skin, to use facial cleansers with a neutral pH level that won't dry out the skin or alter its pH level.

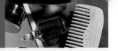

Your Skin Will Age

There is some consolation: Already, the aging of the skin can be halted or delayed to a certain extent. Basically, the aging of skin is due to the same causes that affect all the other organs and metabolic processes in the body. The supply of nutrients to the cells deteriorates, and waste products aren't transported away as effectively. Cell division has slowed down, and more cells die. Tissue fibers, just like muscles, are subject to this natural process of wear.

Reliable from Birth to Old Age

Even if you are sometimes unhappy with your skin, remember that, as a rule, it copes with everything that you subject it to throughout your life. It grows with you, and it expands or shrinks down if you gain or lose weight. It fulfills all its functions even when you are very old. But what concerns many women is the appearance of their skin. A fresh complexion depends on many processes in all three skin layers. However, the epidermis is at a slight disadvantage. Having no blood vessels of its own, it has to rely on the dermis below for its supplies. Therefore, if the supply of nutrients is disturbed, the epidermis is the first to suffer—and everybody can see it!

The skin surface is one of the human body's most important and life-sustaining organs. Even if only a third of the skin is destroyed—for example, through burns—death will ensue.

How Moisture Is Locked In

Only a few years ago, scientists came upon a process that plays a major part in the moisture balance of the skin. Without it, the collagenous fibers couldn't store nearly as much moisture as they do. The moisture is partly supplied by the metabolism, but the fibers also absorb moisture from the skin surface itself. And this is where scientists discovered certain biochemical processes, which were summarized as "moisture-retaining factors." These are processes on the skin surface that prevent moisture from evaporating too soon. They have become the focus of cosmetic research, which is focusing on how these processes can be stimulated in old age.

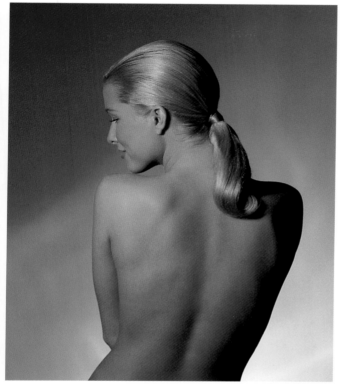

Young, firm, well-moisturized skin develops from the teamwork of many enzymes in the skin cells.

Smoking impedes the blood circulation of the skin and, with it, the supply of nutrients. Simultaneously, smoking impairs the removal of waste products and toxins. As a result, the skin wrinkles prematurely and becomes pale gray in color. British doctors discovered that the skin of women who gave up smoking looked much younger, rosier, and smoother after only one year.

The First Few Wrinkles Are Invisible

Others won't notice for a long time, when a close look in the mirror has revealed to you those fine lines that have suddenly appeared around your eyes and between your nose and mouth. Later come the wrinkles on the forehead. Once you hit 40, however, the characteristic wrinkles around the mouth and on the neck will show your age. Nevertheless, exactly when this aging process begins largely depends on your genetic predisposition and your own lifestyle. Because the first wrinkles usually appear around age 30, it is worthwhile starting to care for your

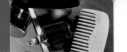

Stress, anger, relationship or money problems? Your mirror will tell you how far these have crept "under your skin."

The Aging Process of the Skin

- The elastic fibers that follow every movement of the body lose some of their elasticity and become stiff and brittle. This explains the formation of wrinkles in the face, because facial expressions cause it to be in motion all the time. These wrinkles will become progressively deeper with age.
- The collagenous fibers also become harder and more brittle, and can no longer store as much water as before. The skin dries out and wrinkles. As if this weren't enough, the number of collagenous fibers decreases with age.
- As with all other cells, the skin cells lose their ability to grow and divide. Consequently, fewer dead skin cells reach the visible surface of the skin, and the renewal process that usually takes about a month in young people will take much longer. The skin noticeably loses its radiance and its rosy shimmer.
- The elasticity of fibers and muscles decreases. With the loss of moisture comes the typical phenomenon of sunken cheeks.

---

skin early on, in order to prevent the formation of deeper lines. And try to avoid creating those worry lines because you're worried about having lines.

What Accelerates the Aging of the Skin?

1. Your overall lifestyle: What is meant here is a poor, unbalanced diet as well as insufficient sleep and exercise. A moderate and sensible lifestyle will help to delay the aging process all around.
2. Stress: It causes the increased release of the stress hormone adrenaline, which damages the fine blood vessels on the skin surface. These blood vessels will narrow, jeopardizing the supply of nutrients. The stress hormone cortisone leads to the formation of fewer collagenous fibers and causes cells to divide less frequently.
3. Smoking: This is about the worst thing you can do.

Smoking causes blood vessels to narrow and aggressive free radicals to develop, which will damage the blood vessels. Nicotine also prevents the absorption of certain vitamins. It is a fact that smokers have a much greater requirement of certain vital substances than nonsmokers. For example, their vitamin-C requirement is about 50 percent higher.

4. Alcohol: Because it puts constant strain on the liver, the skin suffers, as waste products aren't disposed of quickly enough. Alcohol also robs the body of important minerals and vitamins that are essential for healthy and beautiful skin.

5. Environmental poisons: Despite all our efforts, we can't always avoid the harmful substances in our environment. Airborne toxins, harmful chemicals in our homes and at work, as well as many other pollutants can lead to constant skin irritation and the increased formation of free radicals.

6. Sunlight: Both UV-A and UV-B rays cause free radicals to form and initiate biochemical processes that damage

When you have problems, your skin will suffer as well. In some people, it will sag and become gray; others will develop red spots, and still others will acquire skin impurities.

Sufficient and deep sleep is one of the most important beauty elixirs.

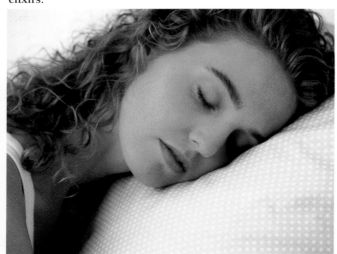

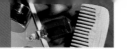

collagenous and elastic fibers. As a result, wrinkles form far earlier than they normally do. Dermatologists refer to this as light aging (as opposed to the normal biological aging process).

7. Weight-loss diets: The quality of the diet is secondary. What causes the greatest harm is frequently alternating weight loss and weight gain, which put a considerable strain on the elastic fibers of the skin.

Prevention or Restoration?

As far as existing antiwrinkle creams are concerned, if you start your wrinkle-prevention program early, you can, with the right creams, face masks, and so forth, increase the skin's defenses against harmful outside influences. Less stress for the skin means better protection for the cells underneath. As a prophylactic measure, cosmetics can also improve the circulation of the skin in general, which in turn will improve the supply of nutrients and oxygen, and this should not be underestimated if you want to keep a youthful appearance. But once wrinkles have formed, externally applied remedies, unfortunately, have little effect.

Tip
Day creams with vitamin A should also contain protection against UV rays. Otherwise, the light would render the vitamin A inactive.

Coenzymes in Skin Creams

Apart from the many plant-based and chemical ingredients, packaging for cosmetics these days frequently lists ingredients such as vitamins, minerals, and trace elements—meaning coenzymes. The immobilizers of free radicals are the most significant—namely, vitamins E and C, beta-carotene (vitamin A in a preliminary stage), and selenium. They actually do influence cell activity in the lower skin layers to a certain extent. Cosmetics may also contain the B vitamins, calcium, and zinc, as well as other coenzymes.

Vitamin A Stimulates Skin Enzymes

More and more cosmetics containing some form of vitamin A are being developed, and these are the ones that are being hailed as the new miracle cures against premature aging of the skin. Trials have actually shown that the depth of skin wrinkles was reduced by 40 percent if a vitamin-A skin cream was used. After only 15 days, the skin was also more elastic. Experts think that enzymes are responsible for this astonishing result, as the additional supply of vitamin A encourages enzyme activity. The epidermis thickens, and the collagen content of the skin increases. This helps UV-damaged skin to regenerate and protects it effectively against renewed UV attacks.

Panthenol for Skin and Hair
Panthenol is nothing more than the well-known vitamin and coenzyme pantothenic acid in a preliminary stage.

Cosmetics that contain enzymes and coenzymes (vitamins and minerals) help to maintain healthy, beautiful-looking skin.

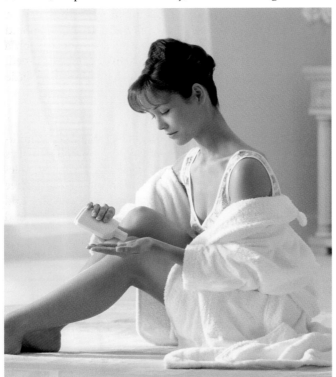

Tip
There is hardly any other factor that accelerates skin aging as much as UV radiation. Moreover, if you decide at age 30 that you should stay out of the sun, it is already too late. As far as skin aging is concerned, the decisive factor is the amount of time you spent sunbathing in your youth. And the more sunburns you have suffered, the greater the risk of skin cancer.

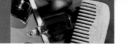

This coenzyme has a central function in the metabolism of each individual cell. Cells cannot survive without it. If there is a panthenol deficiency, skin damage will soon result. It is therefore not surprising that many doctors apply pantothenic acid externally on wounds, burns, and skin allergies. These days panthenol can be found in many day and night creams, suntan lotions, and other body-care products. Even healthy skin can benefit from the enzyme-activating effect of panthenol, as it will stay supple, small wounds will heal faster, and the top skin layer will renew itself again and again.

If your hair has been damaged by perms, has become porous through bleaching, or has split ends, panthenol can also help. Not only can it be found in some shampoos and conditioners but also in certain hair mousses and hair sprays. Exactly how panthenol repairs hair is not yet fully understood. But we do know that it penetrates the hair and binds moisture, making hair more elastic. It also travels to the hair roots where it is converted into pantothenic acid. Scientists haven't thus far been able to establish clearly whether or not it is the enzyme-activating influence of the coenzyme that plays the deciding role in bringing about healthier, shinier hair.

If you want to really pamper your skin, don't just use enzyme-enriched cosmetics, but take enzyme tablets as well.

Vitamin E Controls Important Skin Enzymes
Unfortunately, if the skin is exposed to too much sun, it reacts and can form harmful enzymes. This is where vitamin E comes in. Unlike many other vitamins, vitamin E doesn't work together with the enzymes, but can neutralize the harmful effects that some enzymes have. You can benefit from this if you are planning to sunbathe. You should regularly apply a skin cream with 2.5 percent vitamin E for about 10 days before you intend to lie in the sun. This way, your skin will be so rich in vitamin E that, for instance, you will only need a suntan lotion with SPF 2 instead of SPF 4. If you have already gotten a sunburn, then vitamin E can effectively reduce the pain and inflammation, because it blocks harmful enzymes that normally would only make the inflammation worse. What's more, vitamin E encourages the restoration enzymes in the skin

to work their hardest. Thanks to vitamin E, wounds will heal faster, connective tissue will retain its elasticity longer, and unpleasant brown age spots on the skin will partly disappear.

Enzymes—a New Wonder Treatment for Wrinkles?

Creams, lotions, gels, and emulsions that contain enzymes have existed for some time now. Enzymes can be found especially in natural cosmetics made of plant extracts. Yet their existence there is more or less coincidental. In order to produce an enzyme-specific effect, it is not enough to use these by-products. However, dedicated enzymes are cultivated in laboratories by some cosmetics firms. They appear to be derived from special microorganisms that mainly live in sulfuric thermal springs.

SOD—the Enzyme Formula for Skin Protection

Some beauty-care products for more mature skin already contain the enzyme SOD, or superoxiddismutase. This tongue-twister of a name represents an enzyme that the body produces itself. It provides protection against harmful free radicals from environmental poisons or from strong UV radiation. These damaging substances are thought to be responsible for the formation of premature wrinkles and for early aging of the skin. By adding the SOD enzyme to cosmetic products, it is hoped that a more direct protection of the skin can be achieved. Often cosmetics manufacturers also add the coenzymes of SOD to their products, especially vitamin E, which increase the protective effect of SOD significantly.

A Well-Kept Secret

Cosmetics companies are reticent about what cosmetic enzymes will be able to achieve in the future. Judging by their known properties, however, cosmetic enzymes might be able to strengthen the defensive mechanisms of the skin, thereby protecting it from many harmful influences such as sunlight, environmental poisons, and disease-causing germs. They could also improve blood circulation

Tip
Natural cosmetics that don't contain any preservatives should be kept in the refrigerator. The same goes for all cosmetics that contain enzymes, because they are heat-sensitive.

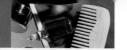

in the skin and thus the supply of oxygen and other nutrients, lending the skin a more beautiful appearance all around. In addition, it is conceivable that enzymes could protect and repair both collagenous and elastic fibers, bringing us an important step closer to the aims of these skin-care products.

Enzymes against Cellulite

Today, there are also enzyme-enriched anticellulite creams on the market. These cosmetics contain active fat-splitting enzymes that are produced according to the most up-to-date biotechnological processes. They have exactly the same structure as the body's own, natural, fat-splitting enzymes, and they are designed to stimulate the breakdown of fat in the tissue. Some of the new anticellulite creams also contain substances that encourage the enzymes that work in the fat cells to do their best, while blocking those enzymes that are responsible for the storage of fat. The manufacturers of these anticellulite creams claim that the skin will become firmer, smoother, and more elastic. However, they also point out that plenty of regular exercise will encourage the body's production of its own fat-splitting enzymes. Don't just trust in synthetically produced enzymes struggling through to the fat cells from the outside, but also rely on your own enzymes, which you can activate with a special anticellulite exercise program.

Recent statistics show that 80 percent of women have cellulite. This weakness of the connective tissue can be traced to genetic and hormonal causes. Therefore, enzymes alone won't defeat the condition—exercise and a low-fat diet are just as important.

Enzyme Therapy Quick Reference Guide

What follows is a quick reference guide in which you will find the answers to the most frequently asked questions about enzymes: Against which complaints are they helpful? For which conditions are they not advised? And when is it necessary to consult your doctor?

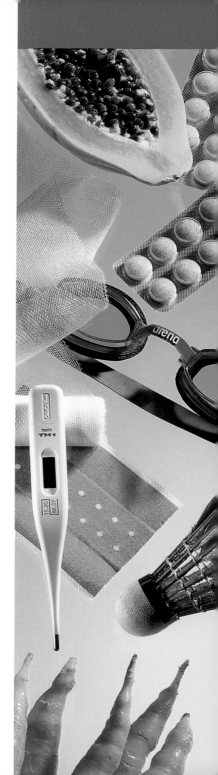

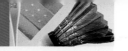

A
Adnexitis
This is the Latin term for inflammation of the ovaries and the fallopian tubes. These inflammations can take a long time to treat, and they may be recurring. There is also a risk that sterility may ensue. Enzymes can support conventional medications and help to prevent sterility. The condition must be treated by a doctor!

Aging
In the biological aging process, all metabolic processes slow down, cells die, and signs of wear and tear become apparent. A course of enzyme preparations should be taken twice a year to improve circulation and boost the immune system. Enzymes also help to prevent heart and circulatory disorders, and are beneficial for many age-related illnesses. As a prophylactic measure, self-medication with enzyme preparations is advised. If you fall ill, however, you must consult your doctor.

Alcohol is one of the enzymes' greatest enemies. However, a glass of wine or a couple of glasses of beer a day are permissible.

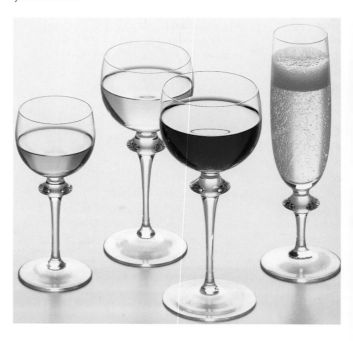

AIDS

All that can be said so far, after careful consideration, is that enzymes may be able to extend the time span between the infection and the outbreak of the disease. Enzyme research in this area still has a long way to go.

Alcohol

With regard to enzymes, alcohol is dangerous because it destroys minerals, meaning vital coenzymes. In addition, alcohol abuse makes excessive demands on the enzyme production of the liver.

Arteriosclerosis

Deposits on the walls of arteries and veins can impair blood circulation and, at worst, block an entire blood vessel. Enzymes have both prophylactic and therapeutic uses, as they are able to remove blood clots that have already attached themselves to the wall of a blood vessel.

Risk factors that encourage arteriosclerosis: smoking, obesity, diabetes, stress, high blood pressure, high cholesterol levels

Arthrosis

One of the rheumatic disorders, arthrosis is caused by wear of the cartilage in the affected joint, and must be treated by a doctor. Enzymes cause the inflammation and swelling to die down and thereby help to lessen the pain, which can sometimes be considerable.

C

Cancer

So far, scientists are more or less guessing as to the effects of enzymes in the treatment of cancer. It is certain that enzymes are beneficial in the aftercare, in order to strengthen the patient's immune system, which has been weakened by traditional cancer therapy, and to improve the patient's overall well-being. Enzyme therapy should be attempted if only for the reason that it has no side effects and can alleviate accompanying side effects of traditional therapeutic methods. It also improves the efficacy of conventional treatments. In addition, enzyme therapy is useful in aftercare following the surgical removal of a tumor.

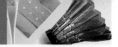
Circulatory Problems

Circulatory problems occur when it is no longer possible to pump the required amount of blood through the blood vessels. The cause is either blood that is too thick or blood vessels that are narrowed or clogged as a result of deposits. In both cases, enzyme therapy is highly effective.

Cystitis

As with all other inflammations, enzymes are highly effective in treating cystitis. If it's just a mild case, then enzymes might suffice as the only treatment; in more severe cases, they can at least be taken to supplement conventional medicines prescribed by your doctor.

Cysts

Cysts can occur in many places in the body. In women, they often show up in the breast tissue, causing pain due to tension. When enzyme preparations are taken, cysts shrink in most cases and sometimes even disappear altogether.

D
Diet

Diet plays a central role when it comes to enzymes. It supplies the nutrients (substrates) that the enzymes require for their work in the body. It also furnishes the body with coenzymes, without which the actual enzymes could not do their work. Coenzymes (meaning vitamins, minerals, and trace elements) are contained in many foods, but they are partly destroyed if foods are stored for a long time, washed excessively, or heated. Raw fruit and vegetables contain the highest amount of coenzymes.

E
Embolism

An embolism is a "migrant" blood clot that becomes stuck in a blood vessel. At worst, it can result in a life-threatening condition if the blood clot causes a pulmonary embolism, a heart attack, or a stroke. Patients need to be treated in the

People spend a great deal of money on medications that improve circulation.

One in 10 people today suffer from bladder and urinary tract infections.

Cysts of varying sizes can be found in about 90 percent of women.

Vitamin-rich fruit activates enzymes.

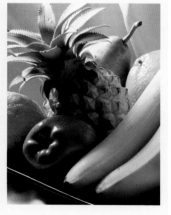

hospital, where they are given powerful enzyme medications that dissolve the blood clot.

Environmental Poisons

Environmental poisons impair enzyme activity in the body in many ways—for example, by overtaxing the body's defenses and encouraging the formation of free radicals.

F

Fitness

Physical exercise is important for enzyme activity, because it improves all metabolic processes and protects against many illnesses. If you keep fit, you will make life easier for your enzymes, and they will thank your body for it with increased activity.

If muscles are tensed, there is a measurable increase of enzyme activity in the blood.

Exercise provides a fitness program for your enzymes.

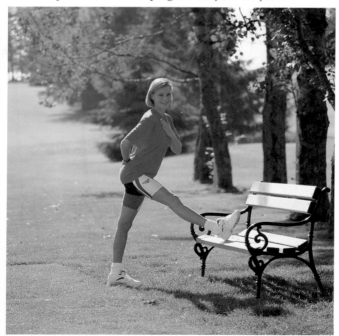

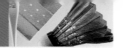

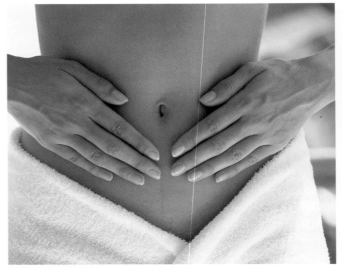

Enzyme preparations that contain mainly pancreatin, an enzyme produced by the pancreas, will help alleviate flatulence.

Tip
Damage from free radicals can be greatly reduced by taking vitamins A, C, B1, B5, B6 and the bioflavonoids, the minerals zinc and selenium, and cysteine, which is an amino acid.

Flatulence

This is one of the many digestive complaints, but it can also occur if you start to include more fiber in your diet. Enzyme preparations will improve digestion. If the complaint persists, you should speak to your doctor about possible causes.

Free Radicals

Free radicals can cause severe damage to cells and are considered responsible for the mutation of healthy cells into cancerous cells. They are produced from environmental poisons, ozone, and aggressive UV radiation, as well as from nicotine and stress. The effects of free radicals are neutralized most efficiently by the body's own enzymes and certain vitamins.

G
Gout
Gout is a condition that is characteristic of an affluent society. It is caused by consuming too much rich food and alcohol. Enzymes are powerless against this illness—only a strict diet can help.

H
Heart Attack
A heart attack is caused by a blockage of the coronary blood vessels either by a blood clot or by deposits in the blood vessel itself. Enzymes are given to treat this condition, but they must be very powerful preparations prescribed by a specialist.

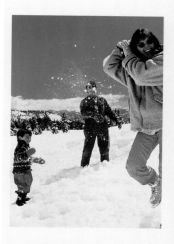

If you are armed with enzymes, you won't have to fear a wave of influenza in the winter.

I
Infections
Enzymes are useful against all sorts of infection, from the common cold to vaginal infections. They stimulate the body's defenses and its powers of self-healing. If you want to protect yourself against infections, you can take enzymes as a prophylactic measure.

Inflammations
Enzymes can almost be regarded as the classic treatment for inflammations. Both on their own and supporting conventional medicines, they help to supply the affected tissue with the necessary nutrients and remove waste products, and they improve circulation and alleviate swelling and pain.

Inflammatory Bowel Disease
In a number cases, enzyme therapy was able to significantly improve the well-being of patients suffering from chronic inflammatory bowel disorders such as Crohn's disease and ulcerative colitis. Sometimes the treatment took the form of enzyme suppositories. However, you should not begin any enzyme therapy without your doctor's consent.

Injuries

With injuries of any kind, enzymes can display their full range of beneficial powers. They accelerate the healing process, help to reduce swelling and inflammation, and cause bruises to disappear quickly (or prevent them from appearing in the first place). In the case of an injury, it is always a good idea to take enzymes.

M
Mastopathy

Mastopathies are benign changes to the female breast tissue. Once the diagnosis has been confirmed by a doctor, enzyme therapy can help to make the lumps disappear within a matter of weeks. However, it's always important to seek medical advice to be sure that the changes in the breast tissue are of a benign nature.

Multiple Sclerosis

This disease of the central nervous system belongs to the family of autoimmune disorders. In addition to other treatment measures, enzymes can contribute to extending the phases of remission between flare-ups.

P
Pancreas

Enzymes can help if the pancreas is inflamed or if it is working less effectively as the result of age or having had surgery. Only use enzymes following your doctor's directions.

Polyarthritis, Chronic

An autoimmune disease, polyarthritis is one of the most painful rheumatic disorders there are. Enzymes can, to a certain extent, dissolve the causative harmful immune complexes and reduce swelling and inflammation. With this condition, it is highly advisable to take enzyme preparations in conjunction with conventional medicines, as the enzymes will help to keep their doses as low as possible.

Tip

Sore muscles are caused by tiny internal injuries to the muscles; therefore, enzymes can alleviate the subsequent pain. It is best to start taking enzyme tablets a few days before a competition.

Multiple sclerosis is one of the most widespread conditions of the nervous system. It is especially associated with partial or complete paralysis and muscle tremors.

This will significantly decrease the often severe side effects of traditional remedies.

Prostate Inflammation
Medicine refers to this benign condition as prostatitis. As with all inflammations, enzymes can help to shorten the duration of the condition and cause the pain to die down more quickly.

R
Respiratory Complaints
If the mucous membranes are swollen, an inflammation is present (bronchitis), and a thick mucus is produced, you should treat these symptoms with enzyme preparations after having consulted your doctor.

S
Stomach and Bowel Disorders
The use of enzymes makes sense for many stomach and bowel disorders, but especially for digestive disorders and inflammatory processes. However, always consult your doctor first to establish a precise diagnosis.

T
Tennis Elbow
This is one of the rheumatic disorders characterized by tension and inflammation of the soft parts ("rheumatism of the soft parts"), meaning the tendons and the muscles. The most common cause is repetitive, one-sided movements. Enzymes have shown good results in the treatment of this condition.

Evidence shows that more women than men suffer from tennis elbow.

V
Vein Disorders
Vein disorders include varicose veins, thrombosis, ulcers on the calves, and phlebitis. All vein disorders are caused

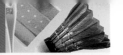

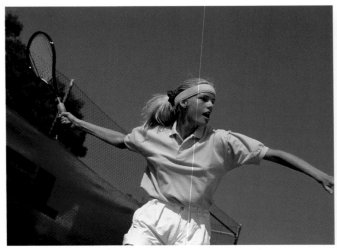

Enzymes will help you recover from a painful case of tennis elbow.

Vitamins work on the cellular level, so a lack of one or several can cause a variety of symptoms.

by a disturbed blood flow, whereby the transport of the blood in the veins back to the heart doesn't take place fast enough. Self-help through exercise, weight loss, and, in some cases, wearing support hose is highly beneficial. In addition, enzymes significantly lessen the symptoms, as they have a thinning effect on the blood.

Vitamins

Vitamins are of great significance when it comes to enzyme activity. Without certain vitamins, enzymes wouldn't be able to do their work. Before enzymes can trigger certain functions in the body, they need a jumpstart themselves. The most important enzyme partners are the vitamins of the B-complex group, including folic acid, biotin, and pantothenic acid. These B vitamins can be found mainly in whole-grain products, vegetables, milk and dairy products, fruit, and lean meat. The vitamins that work together closely with enzymes are also referred to as coenzymes.

W
Weight-Loss Diets

Contrary to popular belief, enzymes can't help you to lose weight, because practically all enzymes are rendered inactive by gastric acid. For this reason alone, it is impossible to eat enough enzyme-rich fruit and vegetables and to stimulate the metabolism sufficiently to cause weight loss.

One-sided diets always lead to deficiencies of certain vitamins and minerals, which in turn disturb the enzyme balance.

Enzyme Preparations at a Glance

Active Ingredients	Indication	Risks and Side Effects
Amino acid hydrochlorides	A mild remedy to support the stomach	In isolated cases, problems of the upper stomach such as stomachache, nausea, and vomiting
Bromelain	All kinds of inflammation coupled with swelling	Allergic reactions, unformed stools; interacts with antibiotics
Bromelain and trypsin	Inflammation of joints, tendons, and muscles, also for edema, injuries, rheumatic disorders, and wounds	Occasional allergic reactions
Bromelain, trypsin, and rutosid	Sports injuries, rheumatic disorders, inflammation of the skin, inflammations in the mouth, the ear-nose-and-throat areas, the digestive and urinary tracts, and the sexual organs	Harmless changes of the stool, feeling of fullness, flatulence; allergic reactions are rare
Fungal enzymes	Disturbed digestion of carbohydrates and proteins; vomiting and diarrhea in infants and toddlers	No known side effects
Lysozym and cetylpyridiniumchloride	Inflammation and infection in the mouth and throat	Hypersensitivity (rare)
Pancreatin	Complaints of the upper stomach, dysfunction of the pancreas, digestive problems without obvious cause, dysfunction of the liver and gallbladder system, feeling of fullness, flatulence	Do not use if you suffer from acute pancreatitis; hypersensitivity, sometimes also of the digestive tract
Pancreatin and dimeticon	Weakness of the pancreas, lack of appetite, feeling of fullness, flatulence, digestive problems after stomach or bowel surgery	No known side effects

Enzyme Preparations at a Glance (continued)

Active Ingredients	Indication	Risks and Side Effects
Pancreatin and fungal enzymes	Digestive disorders; stomach, bowel, liver, and gallbladder complaints	No significant risks are known; do not take if you suffer from fungal allergies or acute pancreatitis
Pancreatin, trypsin, chymotrypsin, bromelain, papain, and rutosid	Inflammation of the skin, the sexual organs, and the respiratory, digestive, and urinary tracts; also for rheumatic disorders and bruises	Color, texture, and smell of the stool may change; allergic reactions are rare
Pancreatin-S	Weakness of the pancreas, liver and gallbladder complaints, cystic fibrosis, digestive problems after stomach surgery, digestive problems due to enzyme deficiency and resulting inefficiency of the pancreas	Do not use if you suffer from acute pancreatitis; in isolated cases, allergic reactions of the skin, nose, eyes, and the digestive tract have been reported
Pepsin and citric acid	Chronic inflammation of the stomach lining due to gastric acid and pepsin deficiencies, stomach-related diarrhea, digestive complaints, anemia caused by iron deficiency	No known side effects; do not use if complaints are caused by excess gastric acid
Rizolipase, fungal protease, and amylase	Digestive problems due to pancreas dysfunction	In isolated cases, diarrhea, nausea, constipation, and upper-stomach complaints have been reported
Trypsin, papain, and bromelain	Inflammation, weakened immune system	Allergic reactions are rare
Trypsin, papain, and chymotrypsin	Supports the treatment of inflammations, viral infections, and cancer	Occasionally, harmless changes of the stool; allergic reactions are rare

The Most Important Enzyme Therapies at a Glance

Condition	What Enzymes Can Do
Arthrosis	Enzymes cannot reverse this condition, which results from wear, but they can stabilize it and alleviate pain.
Bronchitis	Enzymes reduce the swelling in the respiratory tract, make mucus more liquid, and act as an expectorant.
Cancer	Enzymes cannot cure cancer, but they can boost the body's defenses against cancer cells and alleviate the side effects of cancer therapies.
Cystitis	In mild cases, enzymes are well suited to lessen the frequent urge to urinate and to decrease the pain when urinating.
Digestive disorders	Digestive disorders occur when there is a deficiency of digestive enzymes in the body. Enzyme preparations can, to an extent, replace these enzymes and thereby alleviate digestive disorders.
Embolism	In hospitals, powerful enzymes are used to dissolve life-threatening blood clots.
Endometriosis	Enzymes reduce the risk of sterility by causing the scattered fragments of the womb lining to leave fewer scars.
Heart disease	Enzymes improve blood flow, make blood vessels more elastic, transport waste products and deposits away more quickly, and supply the heart with oxygen and nutrients faster.
Infections	Enzymes support the treatment of all kinds of infection. They strengthen the macrophages in their fight against pathogens.
Inflammation of the fallopian tubes	Enzymes prevent adhesions within the fallopian tubes. They also encourage the healing of wounds.

The Most Important Enzyme Therapies at a Glance (continued)

Condition	What Enzymes Can Do
Injuries	In cases of sprains, bruises, and dislocations, enzymes help to alleviate swelling and remove clotted blood by improving blood circulation in the affected tissue. Pain will thus die down more quickly.
Phlebitis and thrombosis	Enzymes improve the blood flow, dissolving even the smallest blood clots, and thereby prevent thrombosis. If a blood clot has already developed, enzymes can dissolve it and reduce the inflammation.
Rheumatic disorders	The anti-inflammatory properties of enzymes alleviate pain, reduce the swelling of joints, and make joints more mobile. Antibodies that have turned against the body by mistake are transported away.
Sinusitis	Enzymes reduce the inflammation and also reinforce the effect of antibiotics that are used in more severe cases.
Tender breasts	Enzymes reduce the painful swelling of the connective tissue.
Toothache	Enzymes support the healing of inflammation in the mouth, particularly after a tooth has been pulled. They prevent swelling of the cheek if they are taken three days before the visit to the dentist. They also guard against pain and inflammation.
Weakened immune system	Enzymes boost the body's defenses and stabilize the immune system.
Wounds	Enzyme creams are well suited for cleaning wounds. They remove damaged tissue and prevent inflammation.

The Most Important Coenzymes in Food: An Overview

Mineral/Trace Element	Deficiency Indications	Important Sources
Calcium	Bleeding gums, aching bones, osteoporosis	Milk and milk products, liver, linseed, sesame seeds, parsley, shellfish, legumes
Chromium	Raised cholesterol and blood-sugar levels	Cheese, sweetbreads, leeks, nuts
Copper	Lack of concentration, reduced ability to retain information	Cucumbers, oysters, fish, nuts, legumes
Iodine	Problems with the thyroid gland	Iodized cooking salt, saltwater fish
Iron	Fatigue, migraines, cracked corners of mouth, lack of concentration	Nuts, millet, legumes, sweetbreads, soybeans, sesame seeds, meats, eggs
Magnesium	Muscle cramps, heart and circulatory trouble, lack of concentration	Cocoa beans (chocolate), nuts, potatoes, green cabbage, peppers, spinach, broccoli
Manganese	Bone and dental complaints	Wheat bran, hazelnuts, oatmeal
Molybdenum	Impotence, gout, kidney stones	Buckwheat, garlic, soybeans, wheat germ
Potassium	Lack of appetite, digestive trouble, lack of motivation, arrhythmia	Whole-grain products, nuts, vegetables, fresh fruit, fruit juices, legumes
Selenium	Lowered resistance to infection, heart complaints, cataracts	Fish, nuts, whole-grain cereal products, sesame seeds
Zinc	Hair loss, skin complaints (eczema)	Meat, organ meats, eggs, seafood, soybeans

The Most Important Coenzymes in Food: An Overview (continued)

Vitamin	Deficiency Indications	Important Sources
Vitamin B1 (Thiamin)	Irritability, loss of appetite, sleeplessness, digestive trouble, edema	Liver, pork, legumes, potatoes
Vitamin B2 (Riboflavin)	General fatigue and listlessness, irritation of mucous membranes, nervous complaints	Meat, saltwater fish, liver, whole-grain products, milk and milk products
Vitamin B6 (Pyridoxine)	Loss of appetite, bowel complaints, skin changes, fatigue	Wheat germ, fish, cabbage, potatoes, legumes
Vitamin B12 (Cobalamin)	Paleness, white lips, burning sensation on the tongue, stomach and bowel complaints	Sauerkraut, liver, milk and milk products, fish, eggs
Vitamin C (Ascorbic acid)	High susceptibility to infections, loss of appetite, easily becoming tired	Potatoes, peppers, kiwifruit, citrus fruit
Niacin (Vitamin B3)	Fatigue, dizziness, headaches, skin inflammation, diarrhea, loss of appetite	Lean meat, poultry, fish, mushrooms
Folic acid	Anemia, sensitive mucous membranes, problems in pregnancy	Cabbage, spinach, carrots, beans, whole-grain products

Index

Index

About the Authors
Friedrich W. Dittmar, M.D.
The head of the gynecological department at the district hospital in Starnberg, Germany, Dr. Dittmar uses enzyme therapy successfully in treating many female disorders.
Jutta Wellmann
A renowned scientific journalist, Jutta Wellmann writes regularly for various magazines and is the author of several health guides.